WHAT IN THE WORLD ARE CT SCANS?

WHAT IN THE WORLD ARE CT SCANS?

Dr. Austin Mardon, Aamna Idrees, Hafsa Idrees, Isra Ziad,
Hannah Nie, Anushka Hasija, Maggie Wang, Alexander Martin,
Tenzin Yehshopa, Hannah Schepian, & Viveka Pimenta
Edited by Taryn Foster

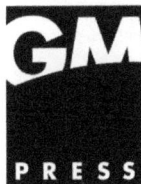

GM

PRESS

2021

Contents

CHAPTER 1

Origins of CT Scans

Aamna Idrees

X-rays

For much of existence, humans have been fascinated by the unseen. Civilizations have taken to studying the mysteries that lie in swaths of space and the depths of oceans. Ironically, for a while the most inaccessible mysteries were the ones closest to humanity, lying below the surface of our own skin. The human body has layers to it much like the ocean, from organ systems to organs to tissues and beyond. The man that first cracked the visual barrier between people and their own biological depth was Wilhelm Conrad Roentgen.

One of the greatest achievements in medical imaging was discovered by accident. Dr. Roentgen was a physics professor in Wurzburg, Bavaria ("Scientist Discovers X-rays"). In 1895, Dr Roentgen performed a study to test if cathode rays could pass through glass. In a surprising twist to his experiment, incandescent light passed through his black paper set up to project onto a fluorescent screen ("History of Medicine: Dr Roentgen's Accidental X-rays"). Thus, the X-ray was discovered. After further experimentation, Dr. Roentgen realized X-rays left shadows of the objects it passed through. Furthermore, the rays could penetrate human flesh, but increasingly dense materials such as bone remained impenetrable ("Scientist Discovers X-rays").

Dr. Roentgen's discovery helped medical examiners make a leap from using invasive techniques in diagnosis to the discovery of all manner of bodily concerns through a screening. X-ray shadows could be photographed and when passed through the human body, one could obtain a clear visual of previously impenetrable inner structures like bones—no surgery required.

While the adverse health side effects of X-rays were a problematic consequence discovered further down the line, that is a topic for another time. Instead, the limitations of X-rays should be touched on as they ultimately led to the need for research and experimentation that ushered in the era of CT scanners.

X-rays were a formidable leap in medical technologies, but they weren't without their shortcomings. While seeing into the human body was a newfound blessing, the resulting 2D images of X-ray scanners felt inadequate at times for understanding an internal issue. Medical professionals needed X-ray images from multiple angles to obtain a more detailed picture of what they were working with (Britannica, 1998). Additionally, X-rays had a density recognition problem. To the X-ray, all tissues were screened equally with disregard to layers of tissues of varying densities (Britannica, 1998). Furthermore, soft tissue diagnosis is not a strong suit of X-rays, leading to difficulty in detecting certain types of injuries such as within organs (Britannica, 1998).

While X-rays were a breakthrough in medical technologies, they certainly were not a solution. The world needed new advancements to fill the gaps between the X-ray's capabilities. Some of the answers were soon to come, in the form of CT scanners.

CT Scanners

Computerized axial tomography scan. Computerized tomography scan. CT scan for short. All are terms used to refer to the same type of medical imaging technique. CT scans elevated the abilities of medical professionals in diagnosing a variety of internal issues within patients. Where X-rays are phenomenal at analyzing bones and joints, CT scans work to fill in X-rays weaker points. Layered tissue and soft tissue analysis were made possible using CT scans ("Differences Between X-rays, CT Scans, & MRI's"). Soft and dense material analysis is not the only area where CT excels, but through the resulting images as well. CT scanners provide more detailed images of internal structures than X-rays, with the ability to deliver cross sectional 3D images of the body ("Differences Between X-rays, CT Scans, & MRI's"). See further chapters for the technical developments and uses of CT scanners.

So how did such a machine come to existence? Certainly, the discovery of X-rays and its subsequent room for improvement led a handful of researchers to explore new and improved possibilities in the world of medical imaging. Tomography techniques have been used in X-ray photography since the 1930s ("Visualizing the Body"), but further research and development of these techniques towards the formation of advanced devices such as the CT scanner were already in motion years prior. Theoretical research into the techniques were published as early as 1917 (Lell et al. 629-644), with the theories and research solidifying greatly over the years and into the 1960s, which saw further publications and the inclusion of hardcore mathematics (Britannica, 1998). The early 1960s was also when the first scanner prototype was built (Mazziotta et al. 169-170).

Researchers and inventors from many parts of the world were on the right track and steadily gaining momentum into the world of CT scanners with their individual efforts. Eventually, the breakthrough was achieved in 1971 when the first functioning CT scanner prototype was used to successfully scan a patient's brain ("Visualizing the Body"). The 1971 prototype did not include computer generated images, and at first there was not a definitive plan to add them ("A Gentleman's Crazy Idea"). When later models of CT scanners would regularly incorporate computers, the X-ray and computer combination would pose as an exhilarating example of the benefits of combined technology for the medical world. The first physical trial of CT scanners set in motion the race for improvement on this novel device. A mere four years later, in 1975, the first full body CT scan was established ("Visualizing the Body"). The world could now move past brain scans and perform all manner of internal diagnostics. Thus, the early 1970s is pegged as the time when CT scans first became available (Britannica, 2012), and they would only increase in popularity and frequency in the years to come.

With a brief timeline laid out, one cannot be reconciled by numbers alone when reliving the origins of the CT scanner. After all, credit should be given where credit is due; who were the key individuals who played a part in the birth of a revolutionary machine? Some names are more highly praised and acknowledged than others. However, each contributor played pivotal roles in the creation of CT scanners. Though many if not all of them worked individually from each other, their individual contributions fuelled the inventive journey and amassed to a truly groundbreaking discovery.

Johann Radon

As with any great invention, the first step is the cultivation of an idea, and a solid understanding of the theoretical workings involved in a target achievement. Even before the creation of a blueprint, one needs to have a clear mental expectation that leads to testable hypotheses. Where then, does the understanding of CT scanners begin?

The answer can be pinpointed to the Austrian mathematician, Johann Radon. Dr. Radon authored a number of research publications. His doctorate dissertation of 1910 was his first published paper, and focused on the topic of calculus of variations, which centers around connections between analysis, geometry, and physics ("Radon, Johann, Complete Dictionary"). With this integrative research background, Dr. Radon went on to form the Radon transformation technique in 1917, which would come as an immense benefit in the creation of CT scanners ("Johann Radon Formulates the Basis for Computed Tomography").

The Radon transform involves some mathematical models which are used to obtain data on a two dimensional plane to create a three dimensional image. The mathematical model allows one to obtain densities of various functions along multiple lines at different angles (Beatty 10). The collective density data is then used in the construction of the image (Beatty 10). While this is a very basic interpretation of a mathematical technique, the mental image elicited serves to explain the important applications of Dr. Radon's model.

An additional display amongst his many achievements was Dr. Radon's demonstration of the creation of a three dimensional object image, which, he reasoned, could be built from an infinite number of two dimensional images of the object ("Johann Radon Formulates the Basis for Computed Tomography"). In other words, the use of multiple 2D representations of an object from various angles could create a 3D model. To visualize this idea, consider a pit inside of a food, for example an avocado pit. In order to view the pit, it would make sense to cut out wedges of avocado flesh in order to expose what is inside. The view from one angle, or one removed wedge, falls rather flat since only one section of the pit is viewable. However, cutting out multiple wedges from different angles will allow you to see within the fruit towards its centre. The more angles you cut from, the better the 3D shape of the pit is exposed. Likewise, the more 2D images obtained from various angles of an object, the better the resulting 3D image will be when compiling all the data. Dr. Radon's demonstration of using two dimensional images to create a three dimensional object image is relevant when recalling the limitations of X-rays. The resulting data image from X-rays is two dimensional, and medical professionals need to view a patient's internal system from multiple angles to obtain a clear understanding of the situation at hand. Using Dr. Radon's three dimensional image construction technique, X-rays may be a part of the solution to their own limitations. Multiple X-ray images, when put together, could render a three dimensional model. This idea would later turn out to be a key process in the functioning of CT scanners down the line of developments.

While he did not know it at the time, Dr. Radon's work would set the course for computer tomographic techniques to take the stage in health care settings. Dr. Radon accomplished a lot of brunt mental work to get the foundations of CT scanners on the table. However, taking a leap from a mathematical model to a physical invention is no minor task. So while research is integral to societal advancement, it is equally pertinent that theoretical workings be applied to tangible models to legitimize or advance existing knowledge. Therefore, the transition from paper to parts must be made. Parting ways with the critical feats of an Austrian mathematician, the focus now goes to the birthplace of such a transition: at the hands of an American neurologist.

William Oldendorf

While Johann Radon started the theoretical foundation for CT scanners, the medical imaging world had yet to see ideas manifest into a physical representation. The credit for breaking the barrier between research papers and a working device falls to William Henry Oldendorf. Dr. Oldendorf was a professor and medical researcher (Baranauckas, 20). Dr. Oldendorf was interested in pursuing new avenues in medical imaging diagnostic techniques due to his distaste in having to perform invasive measures as a clinical neurologist (Greenburg 148-149), and felt that the world of health science could do better in their methods of information collection.

After witnessing an engineer using X-rays to find dehydrated parts of frost-bitten oranges, Dr. Oldendorf looked into radiation absorption patterns as a means to determine complex internal structures of objects (Mazziotta et al. 169-170). Thus, the spark for invention was lit. With household materials, Dr. Oldendorf created a radiograph tomogram using back projection (Mazziotta et al. 169-170). Back projection is one of the earliest and simplest reconstruction methods (Orrison Jr and Sanders). It involves piecing together an object's image using image slices obtained from the passing of X-rays through the object. Dr. Oldendorf's initial design allowed him to research, write, and eventually publish his work on cross sectional brain scans using X-rays— the first of its kind (Baranauckas, 20). His paper described the results of his experiments scanning an object from many angles all around the object's body. Dr. Oldendorf's demonstration provided theory for the creation of cross sectional images of the head using slight density variations of internal structures.

He was also the first to obtain a patent for creating an advanced scanner in 1963 and worked independently to build the prototype through the early 1960s (Mazziotta et al. 169-170). The device he crafted had a transportable energy-rich photon source and a mechanically coupled detector (Baranauckas, 20). Photons are elementary particles that make up light, and can also be described as composed of electromagnetic energy or radiation (Puiu). Photons have energy, but are not charged and have no mass (Puiu). The detector was a recording medium to catch the X-ray images and visualize them.

Undoubtedly, Dr. Oldendorf's machine held exciting implications towards practical uses in diagnostic imaging. His inventive streak was not a stranger to hurdles, however, as the gateholders to further, more large-scale production did not share similar enthusiasm. Many major X-ray manufacturers were uninterested in taking on his invention due to failure in recognizing the potential market for a device that they thought had a limited and trivial purpose, with high production costs to boot (Wolpert 605-606). Facing a lack of commercial funding, Oldendorf was unable to further his design. However, the torch to CT scanning production was going to pass on to another individual, who would go on to recognize Dr. Oldendorf's work in his own publications as he brought CT scanners to public light. Before jumping from one inventor to another, there is more theoretical foundation to be explored, contributed by South African American physicist Allan Cormack.

Allan Cormack

Though research and development on CT scanners was steadily gaining ground, Allan MacLeod Cormack may be a prime example of jumping on the CT bandwagon a little early. His enthusiasm for research in the topic of CT scanners was a good thing though, as his findings proved important in obtaining a comprehensive understanding of the capabilities of CT scanners and improving future models. Unlike Johan Radon, whose applicable theoretical work stemmed from his doctoral studies, professor Cormack tinkered in CT scanning experiments during his spare time. At first, when professor Cormack published his papers on CT scanners in 1963 and 1964, he received virtually no audience interest in response (Allan M. Cormack – Biographical). It appeared that, continuously, interest in CT scanners was born in each individual contributor to the topic, but subdued with them as well due to poor reception. Therefore, though the topic of CT scanners was not necessarily novel during professor Cormack's time, it was still very much alien to the larger body of researchers.

Professor Cormack's papers, which were published in the Journal of Applied Physics (Tan and Poole, 4-5), provided a much needed theoretical basis on the concept of computer tomography. His studies resulted in the development of the mathematical technique behind CT scans (Wolpert 605-606) ; in other words, a model outlining the formation of three dimensional images through the culmination of X-ray data taken at multiple angles. The technique was discovered when professor Cormack moved an X-ray source and electronic detectors around a specimen of interest (Britannica, 1998). The data from this procedure was obtained and underwent computer analysis, which revealed the creation of a detailed image of tissues in the cross section of his specimen (Britannica, 1998). The key to soft tissue imaging was revealed in professor Cormack's hands-on experiment, and he immortalized the procedure in mathematics to the benefit of future researchers, and humanity as a whole.

Although professor Cormack's findings did not gain popularity at the original time of publication, they would not go unnoticed. It would be some years later, from 1971-1972 when the first successful, patient-tested CT scanner was born and brought public attention, that professor Cormack's time for recognition would come. In fact, he would go on to be awarded the 1979 Nobel Prize in Physics for his outstanding work in the field of computer tomography scanners (Vaughan). He shared this prize with another major contributor to the field: Godfrey Newbold Hounsfield. Interestingly, Allan Cormack and Godfrey Hounsfield worked independently from each other (Britannica, 2012). Dr Hounsfield was unaware of professor Cormack's work, and it was Cormack who found out about Hounsfield's successful commercial scanner (Vaughan). The news brought professor Cormack back into the thick of CT scanning action as he dedicated more efforts to researching the field in light of rapid acceptance and development of the machine (Allan M. Cormack – Biographical).

At last, CT scanners see commercial success and are met with widespread enthusiasm by scientists, medical professionals, X-ray developers, and the general public. This long-awaited step into fame can be credited to an English electrical engineer.

Godfrey Hounsfield

Godfrey Newbold Hounsfield was an English electrical engineer who created and tested the first commercial CT scanner in 1971. Hounsfield worked independently to manufacture a CT scanner that was tested on October 1st, 1971 at the Atkinson hospital in Wimbledon, London ("A Gentleman's Crazy Idea"). Dr Hounsfield was in the company of radiologist James Ambrose, whose 41 year old patient (Lell et al. 629-644) had a suspected brain tumor and was serving as a trial subject ("A Gentleman's Crazy Idea"). Dr Hounsfield's machine scanned the brain of the patient, and when data from the scan was collected and compared with the results of the surgery Dr Amborse performed, both men were joyfully astonished. The resulting three dimensional image of the patient's brain, obtained from the CT scan, revealed a tumor-like mass that was very similar in shape to the mass that was removed during surgery (Wininger). Not only that, but the CT scanner's images were incredibly detailed; Hounsfield and Ambrose could make out the cortex, cerebral spinal fluid, and white matter in the brain ("A Gentleman's Crazy Idea"). Thus the CT scanner saw its first success in health care.

As mentioned early in the chapter, the first clinical model of the CT scanner did not have an incorporated computer, and there were initially no plans to include one ("A Gentleman's Crazy Idea"). Instead, Hounsfield took the data from his scanner, which was stored on a magnetic tape, to the EMI (electric and musical industries) lab for analysis ("A Gentleman's Crazy Idea"). Housnfield and Ambrose published the results from their first test on April 20, 1972 ("A Gentleman's Crazy Idea"). Their clinical trial would go on to encourage the production of CT scanners and eager incorporation of the divide in medical settings and beyond. Soon, computers were integrated into the machine's design. CT scanners were no longer a wild idea, but a great technological achievement.

Conclusion

The journey retracing the origins of CT scanners comes to a close. The story is as unique as the machine itself. Five men and their accomplishments, and likely countless other unsung contributors are threaded together in the narrative. Each of them is part of the same grand story, though none of them knew they were playing critical parts at the time of their discoveries. The diversity of individuals in terms ethnic background and profession speaks to humanity's ability to achieve the seemingly far fetched and impossible when united through common goals and interests.

The origins of CT scanners are, unsurprisingly, just the beginning. There are many more aspects of this now essential device to be explored. For example, how exactly did Godfrey Hounsfield achieve what some researchers before him failed to achieve by garnering public interest in CT scans? How important are these devices in medical diagnosis, and some may be wondering what even are CT scans and wish to dive in more detail regarding the machine itself. Furthermore, there may be questions as to how far research into CT scans has progressed in the modern day; do we know everything there is to know about these machines? From CT scanners roles in everyday medicine to the use of CT scanners for children, many topics will be discussed in further chapters.

In the next chapter, one last trip in the past awaits to explore in more depth the life and accomplishments of Godfrey Hounsfield, the man who took the world by storm with the first creation of commercial CT scanners.

CHAPTER 2

The invention of Godfrey Hounsfield

Hafsa Idrees

A Recap of the Origins of the CT Scan

The scientists of the past have played a pivotal role in the contribution of the development of the CT scan. Johann Radon, William Oldendorf, Allan McCormack, Godfrey Hounsfield, and countless forgotten scientists have realized a dream once impossible. Their individual efforts put together a revolutionary machine that changed the field of radiology itself. However, although each individual played their part to fit the key into the lock, one key individual was brave enough to actually materialize the dream into reality, from theory into practice. This leap of faith set this individual apart from the others; while others contributed to the theory of CT scans, proving that it could be made possible, albeit difficult, he was the one who took a step into the unknown and proved to everyone that dreams can be made reality.

One might be thinking, who exactly is this person, and what was so special about this individual that he managed to do what others could not? Well, the short answer is, nothing really. He was not known for being extraordinarily intelligent, nor did he have any noteworthy accomplishments in his early life (Bhattacharyya 448-450), as it is with most prominent individuals in the field of science. However, this individual was notoriously curious. He would experiment with theories of science, often exploring these theories to see if they are really how scientists have explained. This man was an English electrical engineer who employed the help of two radiologists to realize his dream of creating the CT scan (Bhattacharyya 448-450). He was a simple, modest, and well-liked individual, often conferring advice upon his younger colleagues (Bhattacharyya 448-450). Now that the cat is out of the bag, let's take a closer look at this famed individual who revolutionized the field of radiology and medicine through the groundbreaking discovery of the CT scan.

Who was Godfrey Hounsfield?

The man behind the life-changing invention of the CT scan, which changed the world of medical science forever, was none other than Godfrey Newbold Hounsfield, also known as Godfrey Hounsfield. Godfrey Hounsfield was born in 1919 as the youngest of five siblings, in the small town of Sutton-on-Trent, located in the country of Nottinghamshire, England (Bhattacharyya 448-450). As a child, he was known to experiment with theories of science, often encountering near-death experiences due to his dangerous antics. These antics included near-self-destruction when lighting tar barrels in presence of acetylene to see how high they would launch into the air (Bhattacharyya 448-450). He attended the Magnus Grammar School but did not show much excellence in any subject except for mathematics and physics (Richmond 687). He later enrolled into the Royal Air Force right before World War II began, learning electronics and radar science. After the end of the war, Air Vice-Marshal Cassidy, who worked with Hounsfield, was so impressed by his knack for electronics, that he arranged for him to study at the Faraday House of Electrical Engineering by providing him with a grant (Bhattacharyya 448-450). This was the turning point for Hounsfield, as his knowledge acquisition at the college helped him tremendously in developing the CT scan machinery. Perhaps if it was not for Air Vice-Marshal Cassidy, we would not have had the revolutionary technology of the CT scan by Hounsfield.

After graduating from college, Hounsfield joined Electric and Musical Industries (EMI Limited), and was employed there for the rest of his working life. It was at this very company, where Hounsfield worked, that the magic happened. One of his major accomplishments while at the company was helping to create the first all-transistors computer in Great Britain (Bhattacharyya 448-450). Over time, however, Hounsfield's capabilities were questioned by his employers, as they gradually started losing interest in his projects, as it happens with most distinguished personas. One fateful day in the year 1967, however, changed his destiny forever, when he mentioned to his company how he was thinking about building a machine that would help medical doctors see the inside of the human body by compiling X-rays of various angles, forming a 3-D image. The company was quite intrigued by his project idea and granted him permission to pursue the project, believing in the potential this machine could carry. He enlisted the help of two radiologists, James Ambrose and Louis Kreel, to help him understand the fundamental basics of radiology while providing specimens for testing (Bhattacharya 448-450). The device was built, and the first object of experimentation was a preserved human brain. Afterwards, a fresh cow brain from the butcher was procured and also examined using the developed machine, and finally, in true scientists' fashion, Hounsfield volunteered himself as the first live specimen (Richmond 687).

As the success of the machine skyrocketed, it was placed at Atkinson Morely's Hospital in Wimbledon in 1971. It was at this very hospital that the machine Hounsfield created with Ambrose and Kreel was put to the test. A patient at the hospital had a suspected brain cyst, but the exact location of the cyst within the brain was unknown. The CT scanning machine was used, and lo and behold, the physicians could clearly see where the cyst was located (Bhattacharyya 448-450). This was a huge success for Hounsfield and the radiologists, as the results proved that the CT scan machine will be an indispensable piece of technology for years to come, replacing more invasive, and often dangerous, procedures. Hounsfield continued to improve and expand upon the potentials of this technology, by aiming to decrease radiation levels and improve accuracy. He spent the rest of his life continuing the advancement of the CT scan machinery, as well as expanding into the field of nuclear magnetic resonance, which is now known as magnetic resonance imaging.

Hounsfield received numerous accolades for his discovery and development of CT scan machines, the most prestigious of which is the Nobel Prize for Medicine, awarded to him in 1979 alongside Allan Cormack, who also had worked on a similar project and discovered a technique called the radon transform. He also received the MacRobert Award, the highest honour which is conferred upon an engineer, the Lasker Award, Commander of the Order of the British Empire, and elected Fellow of the Royal Society (Bhattacharya 448-450). He was also knighted in 1981, two years after receiving the Nobel Prize. Despite all the awards and recognitions conferred upon him, Hounsfield remained a modest and simple man (Richmond 687). He never boasted about any of his work or all the prizes he had received. He was known to be understanding and kind to his younger colleagues, often telling them that they need not worry about exams, as long as they have grasped the subject matter, along with other pieces of advice (Bhattacharyya 448-450). He was quiet, humble, sociable, and well-liked by others. He died in 2004 in a nursing home, alone, due to the progressively worsening condition of his chronic lung disease (Richmond 687).

How did Hounsfield discover the CT scan?
Hounsfield mentioned in his illustrious Nobel Award Address that previous experimental techniques helped him to discover the CT scan. As he worked on different machinery, he realized that X-rays had more potential to convey important information compared to how it was being used currently (Hounsfield 283-290). He wanted to create a machine that would be able to utilize the full potential of X-rays, while being more accurate and sensitive. However, in his endeavours, he recognized that hundreds and thousands of pictures would need to be taken, with an equally numerical amount of equations that would need to be solved (Hounsfield 283-290). This was a daunting task, but Hounsfield knew

that it was doable, albeit ambitious. He employed the use of theories by two prominent scientists. One was a mathematical theory known as the Radon transform, developed by Johann Radon in 1917, and the other was the Algebraic Reconstruction Technique, developed by Stefan Kaczmarz in 1937 (History of the CT Scan).

In order to test whether his theory would work, Hounsfield fashioned a crude form of the current CT scan machine. Low intensity gamma rays were used as the source, a lathe bed for rotation of the source, and detectors as the initial pieces of equipment (Hounsfield 283-290). At first, it took around 9 full days to completely scan an object. This was mostly due to the low intensity gamma ray source, which required more time to scan the object perfectly. 2 ½ hours would go into processing the image, and another 2 hours would go into producing the photograph if conditions were optimal (Hounsfield 283-290). Hounsfield changed the source to more powerful X-rays, which reduced scanning time to 9 hours, a far cry from the previous 9 days the gamma ray source would take. They were finally able to get down to a speed of one picture per day, although they aspired to reduce the scanning time to only a few seconds at a time (Hounsfield 283-290).

Overtime, as the CT scan machinery was improved and adapted to reduce scanning time and increase efficiency, the scanning time was reduced to a few seconds, a triumph for Hounsfield and his team who spent countless hours perfecting the machinery. The journey of developing the CT scan had come a long way from where Hounsfield, Ambrose, and Kreel started from, exceeding their expectations of its success beyond their wildest imaginations.

How important was Hounsfield's discovery to science?

The discovery of the CT scan by Hounsfield was indisputably one of the most innovative inventions to have graced the race of humankind; its accuracy and sensitivity was second to none compared to other techniques. It had become so wildly popular after its invention that by 1980, 3 millions CT scans had been done (History of the CT Scan). This milestone was reached only 9 years after the first CT scanner was installed at Atkinson Morley Hospital. The discovery of the CT scan not only produced a new piece of technology that would be used far into the future, but also contributed a new unit, known as Hounsfield Units (HU).

HUs are an important dimensionless unit used in CT scans. HUs measure radio density in a quantitative manner, using an attenuation of the coefficient of radiation from tissues during development of CT scan images (DenOtter and Schubert). This coefficient is very important, as it provides information about the density of the tissues within the CT scan image. The absorption of the X-rays by the tissues are proportional to its density. HUs are then obtained by linearly transforming the absorption coefficients, which is based on the HU measurements of air and pure water at standard temperature and pressure, -1000 HU and 0 HU, respectively (Hounsfield Unit).

These units are used in a variety of clinical settings with many different applications. For example, CT scans can produce images of bone, which can be used to then measure bone density. In the event of suspected kidney stones, CT scans-produced images can identify the location of these kidney stones, and measurements in HUs can tell us whether the higher density spots are indeed kidney stones or not. As well, physicians can also access fat content in various places of the human body, such as the liver, kidneys, heart, and more. The density of the fat measured in HUs can provide information of the quality and quantity of the fat relative to other parts of the body, and whether the fat is in a normal healthy range, or whether some complications or diseases can arise due to excess fat (Hounsfield Unit).

Thus, it is evident that the discovery of the CT scan advanced medical science in numerous ways. The contribution of Hounsfield and the radiologists Ambrose and Kreel to radiology made a significant impact on the world, as many lives were saved, and will continue to be saved, in the future.

How do CT scans differ from other imaging techniques?

Before the invention of the CT scan, X-rays ruled the world of medical radiology. In 1895, Wilhelm Röntgen discovered X-rays, which soon became the leading tool to see what lies under the skin of the human body (The Eclectic History of Medical Imaging). However, there are limitations of conventional X-ray technology and this is where CT scans dominate the playing field. There are three main limitations when it comes to typical X-ray technology, which Hounsfield discussed in his Nobel Award Address. The first, and most obvious limitation, is the fact that X-ray's produce two-dimensional images which do not correspond clearly to what is contained within a three-dimensional object (Hounsfield 283-290). Traditional X-ray technology, which you have probably seen at a doctor's office at one point, does not differentiate depth within the human body, and as a result, the location of different human body structures within space can be distorted, or difficult to comprehend. In contrast to X-rays, CT scans produce a three-dimensional image of the object being scanned. This allows for greater understanding of bodily structures within the human body in real space.

The second limitation that X-rays pose is the fact that it cannot identify soft tissues within the human body (Hounsfield 283-290). X-rays can only distinguish between bone and air, which can present a difficult situation to medical practitioners in different situations. For example, if X-rays are used to identify a broken bone within the body, it will not be able to identify any major organ tissues or potential tissue damage, which can be dangerous to the patient. CT scans differentiate soft tissues of the human body from bone and air, presenting more useful, and potentially life-saving information for physicians.

The third limitation is that X-rays cannot measure densities of substances through which the rays have passed through (Hounsfield 283-290). Many tissues in our body vary in density; bone, organ tissue, all of these have various density levels which can aid physicians during body examinations. Although X-rays cannot measure density, CT scans are able to measure the densities of different bodily structures, which are reflected in the three-dimensional image.

Interestingly, Hounsfield also worked on other imaging techniques, specifically nuclear magnetic resonance. Nuclear magnetic resonance imaging, also known as MRI, is a technique which utilizes non-ionizing radio waves which affect the spin state of nuclei when a magnetic field is applied (Khurshid and Hussain 259-64). When the nuclei spin returns back to normal, the length of time it takes to do so provides information about the surroundings of where the nuclei resides (Khurshid and Hussain 259-64). This allows physicians to be able to determine the state of tissue within the human body.

So how exactly do MRI's and CT scans differ from each other? Well the first, and most obvious difference perhaps, is the source of the imaging techniques themselves. MRI's use protons and neutrons to measure tissue variation within the body, and the radio frequencies emitted by hydrogen nuclei when transitioning to ground state form the image (Hounsfield 283-290). CT scans use a more conventional source, which are X-rays. Another difference between MRI's and CT scans are the number of variables each technique could detect. CT scans are able to detect only two variables, a major and minor variable. The major variable it detects is density, while the minor variable is atomic number (Hounsfield 283-290). In contrast, Hounsfield postulated that MRI's could perhaps detect more than one variable at a time. By separating the decay rates of MRI's, it was hypothesized that MRI's would be able to show 27 different arrangements of tissue matter, compared to only 9 with CT scans (Hounsfield 283-290). Finally, CT scans have a greater disposition towards identification of fat tissue within the body. Although both pieces of technology can identify adipose tissue fairly well, CT scans are more advantageous to detecting visceral adipose tissue compared to MRIs, as the MRIs tend to underestimate the deposit of adipose tissue compared to CT scans (Klopfenstein et al. 826-830). However, MRI can be used to detect adipose tissue at levels comparable to CT scans.

Although other imaging techniques existed before the development of the CT scan, many of them, specifically traditional X-ray technology, could not compete against the accuracy and sensitivity of CT scans, which undoubtedly puts CT scanning ahead of the imaging game.

Conclusion: How did CT scans change the future of imaging?

For the first time known to humankind, physicians were able to see the soft tissues within the body of a human, something that could not have been seen using traditional X-ray technology. This imaging technique brought forth the accuracy and sensitivity which other imaging techniques could not bring. The invention of the first commercial CT scanner has been accomplished by several known and hidden heroes; each individual played a vital role in bringing all the pieces of the puzzle together.

However, where credit is due, it must be given. Godfrey Newbold Hounsfield was the key to unlocking this chest of secrets, a chest that was filled with mysteries and doubt, wonder and puzzle. If Hounsfield did not take that small step towards realizing his dreams, the world might not be as we now know it. As Neil Armstrong once said in his historic first steps on the surface of the moon, "That's one small step for man. One giant leap for mankind".

CHAPTER 3

Importance of CT imaging in diagnosis

Isra Ziad

CT scans useful for diagnosis

As it will also be elaborated on in the coming chapters, it will be clearly seen how the modern X-ray and CT scans differ in its structure and applications. X-ray imaging occurs as a patient absorbs x rays as it passes through areas of their body, and the quantity of x rays that does so is subject to the quantity absorbed in a specific tissue like a muscle versus a lung (Center for Devices and Radiological Health). Once the x rays leave the individual's body, it associates itself with a detection device (such as an X-ray film) and displays a two-dimensional image (Center for Devices and Radiological Health. What is Computed Tomography?). On the other hand, a computed tomography (CT) scan also occurs through the varying quantity of X-ray absorption by particular tissues, yet produces a different kind of imaging that is known as cross-sectional imaging (portrays "slices" of a body part) (Center for Devices and Radiological Health. What is Computed Tomography?). In comparison to an X-ray, the CT allows for more detail, as it forms a computerized, 360-degree view of anatomical structures which proves them to be an option in emergency situations (CT scan Versus MRI versus X-ray). Presently, many CT scanners are able to "spiral" scan in addition to the standard "axial" mode, and many are capable of imaging various "slices" at the same time. These sort of advancements result in comparatively larger areas of anatomy to be imaged at a faster rate (Center for Devices and Radiological Health. What is Computed Tomography?). The greatest increases in the application of CT scans have been in terms of diagnosing pediatric patients, as well as with adult screenings, and are sought out to continue (Brenner and Hall 2277). The main reason for the increase of CT scan application in children has been due to the decrease in the time required to complete a scan, which has been less than a single second. This rapid duration of the scan has been the source of the termination of the necessity of anesthesia to stop the child from moving during the scan (Brenner and Hall 2278). With this being said, there is a greater degree of accuracy in diagnosing conditions like appendicitis, a greater efficiency in treating head injuries and multiple trauma in the emergency department, and better care of patients with congenital heart disease and others (Frush 24). On the contrary, the assumed increase in CT scanning for adults is to the most extent from novel CT-based screening programs for individuals who are asymptomatic (Brenner and Hall 2278).

What are the commonly ordered CT scans?

The current utilization of CT scans primarily involves the routine diagnostic assessments of the head and trunk (Cervantes 21-1). Author Guillermo Avendaño Cervantes, a specialist in biomedical engineering, writes the book Technical Fundamentals of Radiology and CT where he elaborates on the common uses for CT scans, topics which will be explored in this section. (Cervantes 21-1 - 21-11). He discusses how the first pictures taken of inside the skull through the utilization of a CT scan displayed the lateral ventricles of the brain. This display indicated that the CT scan was a success as it was able to find the location and the consequent displacement. This was the very first image utilizing the CT, with the image taken in 1974. Within a short period of time after, the software enhanced through its continuing complexity and efficacy which advanced the quality of images. More recent images are able to show the distinction between grey and white matter, soft tissues, and details of bones. Today, CT is used to analyze the majority of diseases that need more intracranial (inside the skull) knowledge, like bleeds, obstruction, and different types of tumours (Cervantes 21-2). Having said that, it is needed to diagnose all kinds of brain and head injuries. In addition to the head and trunk, there are three areas or organs of the body in which CT scans are very useful: the chest, heart, and pelvic cavity. Within the chest cavity, studies of the lungs, bronchi, vessels, heart, and breasts can be executed (Cervantes 21-4). Again, through the usage of CT, diseases like pneumoconiosis, asbestosis, or silicosis, which are all lung-related health issues, can be correctly diagnosed (Cervantes 21-4). Cervantes mentions how, in terms of assessing the heart, there can be restrictions on the quality of images due to the movement of the heart, as there are unnatural observations produced as a result. However, by incorporating some specific conditions in terms of such parameters like the scan time and patient involvement to limit movements of the chest area, useful studies can be carried out. The resolution of the CT scan can display changes of the tissue in the heart muscle and can precisely indicate the position of the boundaries between the chambers of the heart (Cervantes 21-7). Additionally, it is helpful to study the dynamics of the images displayed in the sequence it was taken in to examine the performance of the organ more accurately. Cervantes states that the information that can be obtained from this kind of imaging can be used for studies of the structure and functioning of the chambers, specifically measuring the breadth of the ventricular walls which can be used in studies, as well as for diagnostic purposes. Moreover, within the pelvic region, organs and bones can be studied by utilizing CT (Cervantes 21-11). This allows diseases of the bladder, large intestine and testicles, to be accessed, in addition to finding tumors (Cervantes 21-11).

Recent trends of CT usage

Short time after the invention of the CT, it was seen as a crucial tool in trauma care. The vast growth of technology has led to what is known as a "panscan", which defines the combined CT of the head, neck, chest cavity, abdomen and pelvis (Rubin S53). This method has eliminated the troubles of prioritizing a wide-spread range of invasive and non-invasive tests to confirm timely and appropriate care (Rubin S53). Thus, it is not quite shocking that there have been studies showing that the utilization of CT scans has increased in my countries across the world. Authors comparing the use of CT in emergency departments (ED) visits in the United States and Ontario, Canada had compiled insights about the patterns of increase/decrease in the article, Emergency Department Computed Tomography Utilization in the United States and Canada (Berdahl et al 496-494.e3). The type of study was retrospective; it examined ED visits from 2003-2008. The authors utilized the ED data from the National Hospital Ambulatory Medical Care Survey (NHAMCS), a national chart review survey of the visitations to emergency departments in 50 states and Washington, DC (except for military and federal hospitals). In addition to that, they utilized the National Ambulatory Care Reporting System for data analysis of Ontario. The National Ambulatory Care Reporting System has data about the admission-discharge-transfer systems, patient records, and detailed physician notes. For the purpose of this study, the following visit criteria were searched for in the appropriate data sets for both countries: age, sex, triage level, day, the time of arrival, reason of visitation, how long they stayed, household residence, household income, and whether the patient had a CT scan. Any variables that could not be compared between the United States and Ontario, Canada were changed to restrict it to fit the criteria of both nations. The two variables consisted of the reason of visit, and triage score (how emergent the situation is). Common reasons of visits were grouped by placing the visit types into categories, and there was a 3-level triage score (most urgent, urgent, and least urgent) to resolve the previously stated disparities. It was found that the utilization of CT scans had increased in emergency department visits in both the United States and Ontario (Berdahl et al 491). The rate of visits that included CT scanning per year increased in the US and Ontario between 2003-2008; This extracted an annual growth rate of 13% and 10% subsequently (Berdahl et al 488). The authors highlighted that between 2003-2006, the probability of receiving a CT scan during a US emergency department visit was twice as much, compared to Ontario in which it increased by 69%. There were similar outcomes between the subgroups observed (such as between sex, income,visit length, etc); however, the one subgroup that experienced a decrease in the probability of CT usage was those under ten in Ontario (Berdahl et al 490). Berdahl and his co-authors mentioned how it could be suggested that part of the reason for the differences between Ontario and the United states stem from the adoption of technology at an earlier date in the US. It was sought out that the longer the CT had been seen as the first diagnostic test to perform for a particular condition, the rates of CT were closer in value in both places. For instance, the earliest date in which journal articles elaborating CT in the emergency department for headache were released was in the 1970s, and there was just a 45% difference between the US and Ontario (Berdahl et al 492). Although there are many benefits to utilizing a CT scan in healthcare, particularly trauma and in the emergency department, it should not be ordered without giving much thought to how necessary it truly is.

Overuse of scanning? In children?

It is very important for physicians to outweigh the benefits and risk of a CT. CT scans should not be utilized in a manner that it replaces a comprehensive performed history and physician assessment. Uncritical utilization of a CT, or any diagnostic test, would lead to a number of avoidable repercussions. It more so than not, can result in an overuse of CT scanning, ordering of the wrong type of CT, incorrect interpretation of the results, and a delay of crucial treatments to patients with life-threatening conditions (Schwartz 121). Recall that one of the reasons for the significant increase in the use of CT scans has been to diagnose pediatric patients. Emergency room and pediatric physicians now rely on the CT as a crucial component of giving a speedy diagnosis to children in the emergency room. Although there surely are many benefits to the use of CT scans, it can possibly be overused. A study had highlighted the increase in the use of CT scans in pediatric patients who arrived in the emergency room over fourteen years. Within this time, the number of visits that consisted of having a CT scan had increased by a factor of 5 (from 0.33 million to 1.65 million), yet the total number of visits within that time period were relatively constant (Frush 25). Therefore, the growth in the utilization of CT scans resulted from an increased number of uses (Frush 25). This is even more of a concern among children than adults as they are more radiosensitive, and because they have more years of their lives left, meaning more years in which a radiation-caused cancer can form (Brenner and Hall 2280).

What physicians and radiologists can do to decrease the use of CT

The radiation doses to specific organs from any CT study relies on many factors. The most essential are the quantity of scans, the tube current and time it takes to scan in milliamp seconds (mAs), the size of the patient, range of the axial scan, scan pitch which refers to the extent of overlap among adjacent CT slices), tube voltage in kilovolt peaks (kVP), and the design of the scanner (Brenner and Hall 2278).The radiology technician or radiologist controls a great number of these factors (Brenner and Hall 2278). In an ideal world, these conditions would be altered based on the kind of study and size of the patient, yet it is not a universal practice. Thus, the efforts made towards decreasing the dose of radiation to children and adults for that matter, should be given high priority. The Image Gently campaign has given out guidelines to radiology workers on practices they can encompass when imaging a few number of children in a mixed age hospital (Goske et al 273-274). One is to lessen or "child size" the quantity of radiation utilized. They can contact their medical physicist that can assist them to seek out the baseline radiation dose for an adult patient for that specific CT scan. If the doses are higher than what is recommended, other adjustments can be made. On the other hand, individuals can go on the Image Gently Website, and look at the protocols given for children. Fortunately, these guidelines do not associate themselves with the manufacturer of the CT, age of machine, or the quantity of detectors (Goske et al 273).The second being, to scan only when absolutely needed. Increasing the awareness around discussion of the risk versus benefits of a CT scan adds to the role of the radiologist and gives the opportunity of an educational interaction with the pediatrician of the patient, who has specific medical knowledge of the patient (Goske et al 273-274). In addition to the previous two, scan only in the required area of the body. A follow-up CT scan in a child without any symptoms who just so happen to have a lung nodule is unlikely to need their whole chest to be scanned again (Goske et al 274). And lastly, scan once, as multiphase scanning is not generally needed for children. Multiphase scanning usually leads to two-three times the dose in children, and more times than not, does not add any needed information to diagnose the child (Goske et al 274). In regards to the physicians who order these tests, when they are handling a less serious health condition, other kinds of diagnostic methods should be utilized. It may be straightforward, yet it can be difficult to put into practice in settings where there is a high volume of patients, and thus the time spent with patients is limited. An example is renal colic. It is not a condition that is life-threatening and it can be diagnosed with a good amount of certainty, especially when a patient has had renal colic before (Schwartz 121).

The concerns of radiation levels
When ionizing radiation passes through a body or an object, that body or object absorbs the energy. The energy absorbed from being exposed to the radiation is called a dose (Safety Commission). The three terms associated with radiation dose obtained by CT scanning are: effective dose, absorbed dose, and CT dose index (CTDI) (Brenner and Hall 2278). As further elaborated in the article, Computed Tomography — An Increasing Source of Radiation Exposure, authors Brenner and Hall define each of those terms. The absorbed dose is the energy absorbed for each unit of mass. It is measured in grays (Gy), and one gray is equivalent to one joule of radiation energy absorbed for each kilogram of mass. Interchangeable with "absorbed dose", the "organ dose" will to a great extent dictate the level of risk to that organ as a result of the radiation exposure. The effective dose (measured in sieverts [Sv]) is utilized for dose distributions that

are not always the same quantity (applies to CT). It is formulated to be proportional to a general estimate of the severity of harm to the patient. The effective dose enables there to be a rough comparison between varying CT settings, but the downside is it only imparts an approximation of the risk. On the other hand, the CT dose index is valuable for controlling the quality, but is indirectly related to the organ risk. Organ doses obtained from CT scanning are substantially larger compared to other forms of conventional radiography. An example includes a posterior-anterior abdominal X-ray of which has an organ dose of 0.25 mGy (milligray), which is at the minimum fifty times less than the organ dose of a CT scan of the abdomen (Brenner and Hall 2278). To conceptualize the seriousness of the possible risk, the suggested radiation exposure limits can be analyzed. The average lethal dose of radiation that will eliminate fifty percent of the US population in a span of sixty days is approximated to be between 3,500 to 4,000 mSv (milisievert) (Crownover and Bepko 494). Recall that the value of the effective dose is given here as its value, as stated previously, is formulated to be proportional to a general estimate of harm to a person. The U.S. The Department of Energy only allows a maximum of 50 mSv per calendar year for adult radiology technicians and radiologists (a maximum of about 1.3% of the lethal 3,700 mSv) (Crownover and Bepko 494). To compare this value with the average effective dose of radiation of an abdominal series (numerous images of the abdomen using an X-ray) to an abdomen CT, there does appear to be a significant difference. The abdominal series emits an average effective dose of 0.7 mSv, while the abdomen CT emits an average effective dose of 10 mSv (Crownover and Bepko 496).

Dangers of radiation...leads to Cancer?

The biological significance of ionizing radiation, like X-rays, stems from its energetic nature. The radiation is sufficiently energetic that it overcomes the binding energy of electrons that motions around atoms and molecules. In other words, it is able to push electrons out, thus producing ions (Brenner and Hall 2279). Typically for biological materials, the production of hydroxyl (OH-) radicals from the X-ray associations with water molecules is the most recurrent by-product. What these radicals can do as a result, is associate itself with DNA to break the strands, or cause damage to the bases (A-T-C-G) (Brenner and Hall 2279). This is not to say that X-rays cannot cause damage to DNA molecules directly. Fortunately, to the most part the damage is fixed by a variety of systems within a cell; however, if the double-strand of DNA breaks, it is not as easy to be fixed, and an error in repair can result in outcomes, such as point mutations, that associate itself to cancer (Brenner and Hall 2279-80). The effective doses from CT scans are approximated to fall between one to ten mSV. This range is not much different from twenty mSv, which was the closest doses that are assumed to be received by a group of the Japanese survivors of the atomic bombs (Center for

Devices and Radiological Health. "What Are the Radiation Risks from CT?"). These survivors who are assumed to have received doses that are slightly larger than general CT scans have shown to have a quite small, yet an increased risk for developing cancer (Center for Devices and Radiological Health. "What Are the Radiation Risks from CT?"). A CT scan with an effective dose of 10 mSv might be linked to an increase in the probability of fatal cancer of about one chance in two thousand. This can be compared to the probability of the natural occurrence of cancer within the United States population, which is about one chance in five (Center for Devices and Radiological Health. "What Are the Radiation Risks from CT?"). As stated, the risk of obtaining cancer through the exposure of radiation is considerably smaller than the risk of naturally developing cancer. Nonetheless, this small cancer risk from radiation exposure can turn into a public health issue if a large number of people endure an increased number of CT scans with undetermined benefit. The approximated lifetime risk of death from cancer that is linked to one CT scan of the head or abdomen is calculated by adding the approximated organ-specific cancer risks (Brenner and Hall 2281). The organ-specific cancer risks are derived from the value of organ doses (Brenner and Hall 2281). However, the extent to which a person's risk of developing cancer increases or decreases depends on the persons age, sex, and location at which they were exposed to radiation (Center for Devices and Radiological Health. "What Are the Radiation Risks from CT?").

CHAPTER 4

What is a CT scan?

Hannah Nie

Having discussed the invention and history of CT scans, we proceed to describe CT scans in a modern context. CT stands for computed tomography (Rubin S45), and was previously known as CAT, or computed axial tomography (Miñano and Gates). In essence, CT is an imaging technique in which X-ray scans of a sample are taken and processed by computer algorithms to produce high resolution images and analysis of the sample (Waldman 366). CT scans have many applications in a medical setting, allowing for non-invasive yet highly informative diagnoses (Waldman 366).

How do CT scans work?

CT scans take advantage of the ability of X-rays to penetrate various materials without damaging their structure. CT scanners send X-ray beams through the sample being studied, at multiple different angles. As the X-rays pass through the sample, photons in the beams can be scattered or absorbed by atoms in the material, causing the beams' intensity to decrease (Kak and Slaney 114). Different materials interact with X-rays in different ways, allowing different intensities of X-rays to pass through the sample. X-rays exiting the sample can be detected by components of the CT scanner to distinguish the types of materials present in the sample, and where they are located (Waldman 366).

A material's tendency to absorb X-rays can be quantified by its attenuation value (Adams et al. 279). The attenuation value is measured in Hounsfield Units (HU), named after Godfrey Hounsfield, creator of the first CT scanner. Water and air are used as reference materials - their attenuation values are defined to be 0 HU and -1000 HU, respectively (Waldman 366). Materials with high atomic numbers, like bone, absorb more X-rays and have relatively high attenuation values in the range of 250 to 1000 HU. Materials which allow more X-rays to pass through have lower attenuation values, such as fat, whose attenuation value is lower than that of water, at about -100 HU. Additionally, thicker structures absorb more X-rays, while thinner structures would allow more X-rays to pass through (Adams et al. 279).

The X-rays transmitted through the sample in a CT scan would hit a detector which can sense the patterns they produce. The positioning of the X-ray source and detector relative to the sample would vary in small increments in order to take X-rays from many different angles. The results of the scan taken at each angle can be used to generate two-dimensional grayscale images, similar to a regular X-ray scan, which serve as cross-sectional "slices" of the three-dimensional sample (Withers et al. 6). In these images, areas of low X-ray transmission would appear as lighter regions, while areas of high X-ray transmission would appear as darker regions. This is why bones and thicker structures look white on an X-ray scan, while muscles and fat appear to be darker in colour (Waldman 363).

CT combines traditional X-ray radiography with powerful computer algorithms which can compile the many two-dimensional slices of the scan to reconstruct the sample's three-dimensional structure (Waldman 366). The three-dimensional model that is generated is also known as a tomograph, hence the name "computed tomography". These tomographs are composed of voxels: cubic units of volume which are analogous to the pixels that make up an image in two dimensions (Withers et al. 2). The division of the model into voxels is important because as the computer program generates the tomograph, it assesses the values of certain variables within each voxel, which are then used to differentiate the voxels' contents (Waldman 366). As such, the spatial resolution of the CT scan, or its ability to distinguish between small, closely packed details, is affected by the size of each voxel (Withers et al. 2).

CT scanners

CT scanners vary in their construction but typically consist of three main components: the X-ray source, the X-ray detector, and the sample stage (Withers et al. 2), all of which play important roles in executing the steps of a CT scan as previously described.

The X-ray source generates and emits the X-ray photons that are used to scan the sample. Commonly used X-ray sources for CT scanners are vacuum tubes which contain negatively charged filaments and positively charged targets. The filament gives off electrons when heated, similar to an incandescent light bulb. The electrons are subjected to a high voltage which accelerates them to the targets. Interactions between the electrons and targets cause X-ray photons to be released (Waldman 363). Alternatively, synchrotrons may be used as the X-ray source instead. Similar to vacuum tubes, synchrotrons generate X-rays by accelerating electrons, but they achieve this using magnetic effects rather than high voltage. Overall, CT scanners with synchrotrons are more sensitive, producing scans more quickly and at higher frame rates than those using tubes, but they are also more expensive. Most laboratories use CT scanners with X-ray tubes as they are relatively inexpensive, but sufficiently effective (Withers et al. 3).

The X-ray detector senses X-rays exiting the sample. Detectors typically operate by converting the X-ray signal to visible light, then into electrons which can be further processed and interpreted (Withers et al. 3). It should be noted that X-ray sources and detectors can be remarkably sensitive. Changes in temperature, mechanical inaccuracies, and other factors may produce minute changes in the motion of the source and detector which can greatly disrupt the results of a CT scan; as such, the scan conditions must be carefully calibrated (Withers et al. 4).

Lastly, the sample stage is used to hold the object being studied. The configuration of the sample stage varies depending on the setting in which the scanner is used. CT scans of patients or laboratory animals would require scanners with a stationary sample stage, in which the X-ray source and detector rotate around the sample to obtain scans from multiple angles. In other settings, it may be practical to rotate the sample on a spinning sample stage, allowing it to be exposed to a stationary X-ray source and detector at various angles (Withers et al. 2).

Beyond the fundamentals, the principles of CT scans and scanners involve various technical concepts in physics, biology, and more, which will be explored in greater detail in the upcoming chapters of this book.

Applications in medicine and beyond

Different types of CT scans are available for different applications. Conventional CT scans are used for clinical and industrial purposes. In a medical setting, CT scans can use X-ray attenuation to image calcified structures like bones, which have high attenuation values and absorb a significant amount of X-rays (Withers et al. 12). These scans can be used to diagnose and characterize bone fractures and displacements (Rubin S54). Soft tissues and other materials with lower attenuation values may not be adequately detected by a regular CT scan. To increase the contrast of scans and improve the visibility of such materials, contrast agents composed of heavier elements may be applied to increase their attenuation values. Liquid-based contrast agents containing iodine may be used to stain tissues for medical CT scans. Other forms of contrast agents include gases, like xenon, and nanoparticles (Withers et al. 12). Contrast agents and other variations in the CT scan process have allowed for effective imaging of the heart (angiography), brain, lungs, liver, and more. Overall, CT scans are used in various scenarios which require careful imaging of internal tissues, ranging from characterizing injuries and planning surgeries to monitoring strokes and cancer (Rubin S47-S59). The medical applications of CT scans will be further explored in later chapters.

Other types of CT scans include microtomography (microCT) and nanotomography (nanoCT). Both have higher resolution than conventional CT scans and are typically more suitable for imaging relatively small objects (Withers et al. 2). MicroCT and nanoCT can still be used in biomedical applications, but they are not appropriate for studying patients' body parts. Instead, microCT can be used to scan small biological samples such as rodents in the laboratory, tissue specimens isolated from a patient, or deceased fetuses for post-mortem examinations. NanoCT can be used to study biology on a cellular level (Withers et al. 12-13).

The applications of CT scans extend beyond the biomedical field. CT scans have been used to characterize and inspect manufactured products for defects, particularly those that are not visible externally, to help with quality assurance (Withers et al. 10). MicroCT scans can even be used in food science, to examine the structures of food products and how they can affect consumers' experience of their texture - for example, by imaging the porosity of bread (Withers et al. 13). MicroCT also has important applications in material science, allowing for observations of the internal structures of various materials. MicroCT scanners with rapid frame rates can monitor how materials change over time in different environments, or while they are being used for their intended purposes, e.g. as a material freezes or corrodes (Withers et al. 11-12). CT scans can also be used to image paleontological or geological artifacts such as fossils, soil, and rocks. The technique allows researchers to obtain detailed information about the structures of objects which may be difficult to access or study in detail, for example due to their fragility (Withers et al. 13-14). Evidently, CT scans are a versatile technology which can be harnessed for a variety of applications.

What does a medical CT scan procedure entail?

Medical CT scans may be conducted at hospitals or outpatient facilities. The patient may need to remove their clothing and wear a hospital gown. Metal items, such as belts, jewelry, or dentures, may also need to be removed. Lastly, depending on the body part to be scanned, patients may need to fast for the hours leading up to the scan. These preparations are implemented to eliminate any factors that may interfere with obtaining a high quality image from the scan (Mayo Clinic).

If a contrast agent is needed for the scan, it would be administered to the patient through a method appropriate to the body part to be scanned. Scanning of the esophagus or stomach would require oral ingestion of the contrast material in a liquid form. Scanning of the gallbladder, urinary tract, liver, or blood vessels would require the contrast material to be injected intravenously. The contrast material may be administered by enema if scanning the rectum (Mayo Clinic).

During the scan, the patient would lie down on a motorized table which would move them into the CT scanner. The patient may be held in a specific position by straps, pillows, or a cradle for the head, to provide better scans of specific body parts. If the scan is conducted on a child, they may be sedated to prevent excessive movement which may cause blurred scans. The patient may also be required to hold their breath at specific points to provide the clearest scans. The patient would be required to remain lying in the CT scanner for the duration of the scan. The technologist who operates the CT scan can observe and communicate with the patient from a different room. This complete process, including the preparation steps, generally takes about 30 minutes (Mayo Clinic).

After conducting the CT scan, patients who received the contrast material may be required to wait in the facilities for some time to monitor any adverse side effects. Increased fluid uptake may be recommended to help remove the contrast material from the patient's body. The CT scan results are processed and then interpreted by a radiologist. The results are sent to healthcare professionals to be used in subsequent decision-making (Mayo Clinic).

Pros and Cons

CT scans can have a significant impact on healthcare and other sectors. As such, it is important to consider the advantages and drawbacks of this imaging technique in various contexts. In general, CT scans are a non-destructive, minimally invasive way to study samples of interest, which is particularly important for medical applications as this allows structures inside patients' bodies to be examined without harm (Withers et al. 1). CT also offers unique advantages which sets it apart from other non-invasive imaging techniques. As mentioned in an earlier chapter, CT scans provide a more complete view of a sample's three-dimensional structure compared to X-ray scans, which only show two-dimensional images. CT scans have also achieved higher resolution than X-ray scans, imaging samples with greater clarity and detail. Unlike X-ray scans, CT scans can be taken continuously to monitor changes in a sample over time - a unique feature which has been used in research and industrial settings (Withers et al. 11-12). Additionally, CT scans can detect soft tissue injuries which would not be visible in X-ray scans (Fayad).

Magnetic resonance imaging (MRI) is another alternative to CT. MRI scans are conducted by using strong magnets to generate radio waves which interact with protons in the sample. The protons release signals that can be used to identify the type of tissue they are found in. MRI scans have high resolution, similar to CT scans, and can distinguish between different tissues in even greater detail (Fayad). However, MRI scans are not suitable for patients with metal implants, like pacemakers. These devices may experience electromagnetic induction when exposed to the MRI scanner's magnetic effects, and cause severe burns if in contact with the patient's body (Tagell 2570). In such scenarios, CT scans are the safer choice (Fayad). MRI-related burns may also occur due to skin-to-skin contact creating a circuit loop through the patient's own tissue; as such, safe operation of this technique requires careful placement of the patient's body parts (Tagell 2570).

When considering the time and resource requirements of each technique, X-ray scanning is the cheapest and fastest method among the three. CT and MRI both require more expensive and complex equipment that may be less accessible in comparison. Although CT scans take slightly longer to conduct compared to traditional X-rays, they are still relatively quick and can be conducted in about one minute. As such, CT scans are generally still suitable for emergency situations. MRI scans require a longer time to complete - modern MRI scanners have reached scan times of about 10 minutes (Fayad).

A disadvantage of CT scans is that they may be damaging to patients at higher X-ray doses. Although low X-ray doses are typically used for CT, the radiation exposure could nevertheless contribute to adverse effects, such as an increased risk for cancer (Withers et al. 1, 16), which is discussed further in later chapters. The high cost and radiation risks of CT scan have led to concerns about their cost-effectiveness and debate over the necessity of using CT scans for various conditions. This ongoing debate is very pertinent to the healthcare field as medical CT scans are widely used in numerous countries - in recent years in the United States, 245 CT scans were conducted every year per 1000 people in the population (Oren 245). As CT technology evolves and access to this technique grows, it will be important to keep in mind the costs, limitations, and risks associated with CT scans so that they may be used safely and to their fullest potential.

CHAPTER 5

Use in everyday medicine

Anushka Hasija

Now that we've taken a comprehensive look at what CT scans are, the rich history behind their invention, and how they aid in diagnosis, we can examine the use of CT scans in everyday medicine. This chapter will highlight what CT scans are used for (their medical purposes), as well as concerns of overutilization of CT technology in everyday medicine. Furthermore, broad 'categories' of CT scan use will also be established to showcase the imperative role they play in everyday medicine.

What are CT Scans Used For?

As described in previous chapters, a computed tomography (CT) scan uses a combination of X-rays and a computer to generate images of the organs and other tissues. While a regular X-ray orients the viewer as if they were looking through the body, CT scans take 'slices' of the body (i.e. take cross-sectional images which enables the viewer to see inside the body). As CT scans use X-ray technology, dense substances like bones can be identified easily but softer tissues may appear faint in the image. As a result, physicians often order CT scans with contrast (a CT scan along with a special dye injected into the patient) which block X-rays and appear white, highlighting less dense structures such as blood vessels and organs (Cassoobhoy).

As a CT scan provides comprehensive views of 'slices' of the body's organs and tissues, its uses and applications in everyday medicine are enormous — it can detect bone and joint problems, help locate tumours and blood clots, and help visualize internal changes in the body, just to name a few (Cassoobhoy). Furthermore, CT scans produce high resolution, detailed images of the body's internal structures within seconds to minutes. It is thus not surprising that the prevalence of CT scan use has increased exponentially in recent years. In the US, it is estimated that over 70 million CT scans are performed annually, demonstrating the widespread use of this technology (Bosch de Basea et al. 120). Evidently, CT is a very common procedure. Not only are CT scanners found in hospitals across the globe, but also in outpatient offices (Davis and Shiel).

For the purposes of this chapter, 'categories' of the everyday medical uses of CT scans will be established and subsequently examined in further depth. The first category of CT scan use is to aid in diagnosis. When abnormalities (e.g., abscesses, abnormal blood vessels, etc.) are suspected in the body due to symptoms or other tests, CT scans can provide high resolution images of the tissue of interest and thereby confirm diagnosis (Knott and Huins). Moreover, CT scanning technology has evolved to become optimized for viewing specific tissues and organs in the body, generating images of the utmost clarity in order to improve diagnostic procedures. Another category of CT scan use is to guide treatment plans and procedures (e.g., biopsies, surgeries, radiation therapy). Using CT, physicians can identify the location of a particular pathology — such as a tumour, an infection, or a blood clot — and target it. If a tumour develops or a tissue becomes cancerous, a CT scan can pinpoint where a doctor might need to excise a tissue. Additionally, CT scans can guide treatments like radiation therapy by allowing physicians to pinpoint the exact location of a tumour (Knott and Huins). They can also help monitor the effectiveness of treatments like radiation therapy by comparing successive CT scans and assessing whether the tumours have shrunk. Similarly, CT can help monitor the progression of disease too. The last category that will be discussed in this chapter is the use of CT scans to identify internal injuries and bleeding in individuals who have undergone trauma (e.g., a car accident). Since CT scans are relatively quick procedures, as aforementioned, they are ideal for situations in which urgent diagnosis is required. Through their advancements, CT scans are especially useful for assessing head and brain traumas (Cassoobhoy).

Use of CT Scans to Aid in Diagnosis

Through the enhancement of CT imaging, it has become optimized for viewing specific parts of the body and thus helping identify and diagnose pathologies of these organs and tissues. The importance of CT in relation to these organs and tissues will now be examined.

Diagnosis of Bone and Muscle Disorders

As CT scans of the bones can provide a more detailed image of the bone and muscle tissue and bone structure than standard X-rays, they can thus provide more information related to bone and muscle pathologies. CT is commonly performed on the bones when X-rays and physical examination are inconclusive, or to identify the exact location of the injury (e.g., a fracture) once the injury has been identified by an X-ray. CT scans can be used to assess the bones, soft tissues, and joints for damage, lesions, fractures, or other abnormalities ("Computed Tomography (CT or CAT) Scan of the Bones"). A few of the bone disorders that CT scans can frequently aid in diagnosing include: osteoporosis, osteopenia, traumatic fractures, Paget's disease, bone cancers, and bone infections. Additionally, a CT scan can help detect muscle disorders as well, including: sarcopenia, muscular dystrophy, myositis, cancer, muscle sprains or strains, and tendinitis ("Diagnosing Muscle and Bone Disorders With CT Scans").

Diagnosis of Lung Pathologies

Interstitial pneumonia is a rare kind of lung pathology which affects the tissue that surrounds and separates the alveoli in the lungs, thus interfering with effective gas exchange and impeding breathing ("Nonspecific Interstitial Pneumonia (NSIP): What is it, Causes and Treatment"). As interstitial pneumonias often manifest idiopathically (meaning they arise spontaneously, seemingly with an unknown cause) or in association with collagen vascular disease or inhalation exposure, they are among the most difficult lung diseases to diagnose and manage. Over time, continued use and development of thin-section CT scans, in conjunction with studies done by radiologists, pathologists and pulmonologists, have greatly expanded our understanding of what was once oversimplified as pulmonary fibrosis into a variety of interstitial pneumonias (Rubin). The substantial effect that CT imaging has had on the diagnosis of interstitial pneumonia, as well as clinical decision making, cannot be understated. Due to its accuracy in depicting pathology, thin-section CT has replaced surgical biopsy in the diagnosis of several cases of usual interstitial pneumonia. In fact, its scope goes beyond just diffuse lung diseases — thin-section CT is able to assess other airway diseases too, eliminating the need for bronchography as a diagnostic tool. A study revealed that among symptomatic patients with normal radiographs and ambiguous pulmonary function test results, thin-section CT clearly depicted that the patients had emphysema, thereby emphasizing the sensitivity and specificity of thin-section CT as a diagnostic tool for various lung pathologies. As advancements in tools which can effectively characterize pulmonary structure and function occur, thin-section CT is hypothesized to become more widespread and have a greater effect on diagnosing and managing diffuse lung diseases (Rubin).

Diagnosis of Liver Pathologies

The liver is a major site for neoplasms, as both primary and metastatic cancer can originate in the liver. The liver also has a unique structure as it possesses a dual blood supply from both the hepatic artery and portal vein. From previous studies, it was found that most liver tumours derive their blood supply from the hepatic artery rather than the portal vein. Thus, extensive CT scanning techniques were developed in order to highlight the hepatic artery while simultaneously opacifying the portal vein when imaging liver tumours. This technique, termed dynamic CT, involves CT scanning during catheter-directed injection into the hepatic artery or superior mesenteric artery (Rubin). Additionally, CT scans are ordered with contrast using iodine as the dye. During the development of the hepatic dynamic CT scan technique, the efficiency of iodine delivery was maximized via greater control and refinement of the timing and rate of iodine delivery (Rubin). Interestingly, insights into the pathophysiology of the liver were able to drive the innovation in CT scanning technology in this case, thus substantially improving diagnostic procedures.

Dynamic CT unveiled a unique, new view of the liver in which patterns of liver enhancement could be seen. The application of dynamic CT revealed images of the presence of hypervascular lesions, leading to impaired blood flow to the normal liver which could be observed distinctly. This phenomenon was termed transient hepatic attenuation defects. Further developments in CT technology enabled the introduction of modern spiral CT scans, which produces continuous scans of the body rather than individual slices and can rapidly produce 3D and multiplanar images of the body's internal structures. The development of spiral CT enabled continuous, whole images of the liver to be produced, which markedly enhanced the ability of CT to detect hepatocellular carcinoma and other hypervascular liver lesions (Rubin).

Use of CT Scans in Guiding Treatment Plans and Procedures

Prior to the development of CT, the availability of imaging modalities to identify tumours in the body were limited. Soft-tissue visualization was largely not possible, thus in order to diagnose and assess cancer, physicians relied on displacement of radiographically visible structures. Treatment was also administered in the form of exploratory surgery and radiation therapy, which was somewhat imprecise as radiographs were derived from body surface contours and spatial inferences. As a result, upon the development of CT, its earliest applications were to aid in the planning of surgery (i.e., assessing and locating areas of pathology for subsequent excision) and to aid in radiation therapy — the use of CT would allow tumours to easily be pinpointed and subsequently targeted with radiation (Rubin). While most commonly used to locate tumours in the lungs and thus guide the treatment of lung cancer, CT scanning technology can detect neoplasms virtually anywhere in the body. One prominent example is the role of CT in imaging the chest in patients with Hodgkin lymphoma, which is a blood cancer that originates in the lymphatic system. Lymphography, a technique used to image the lymph nodes, was rarely found to be effective in patients with Hodgkin lymphoma, however CT was able to clearly depict not only cancer-ridden enlarged lymph nodes, but also extranodal sites afflicted with disease (i.e., the spleen). This visualization provided by CT is integral in guiding subsequent treatment plans, which usually entails targeted radiation therapy in cases of lymphoma (Hacking and Amini). Furthermore, CT scans can be used in association with other technologies to obtain even greater visualization and clarity in the assessment and management of various cancers. PET scans are able to generate precise images of lymph nodal metabolism, which works synergistically along with the anatomically precise images generated by

CT scans, thus raising accuracy and becoming a suitable diagnostic tool for staging and guiding therapeutic responses for many types of cancer (Rubin).

Use of CT Scans in Traumas

Finally, and perhaps most importantly, the fast, efficient nature of CT scans enables them to be the perfect diagnostic tool for use in emergency events such as traumas. Prior to the widespread use of CT scans and other imaging modalities, a variety of invasive and noninvasive tests were administered to assess and diagnose trauma injuries. As time is of the essence for survival in trauma, modern developments in CT technology have enabled one "panscan" to be taken (simultaneous CT of the head, neck, chest, abdomen, and pelvis) which has now replaced older diagnostic tests (Rubin). Researchers claim that CT scanning is critical in these situations as it dramatically increases a patient's chances of survival. The use of CT scans is primarily advantageous in head and neck traumas, as conventional techniques (including angiography and pneumoencephalography) are unable to provide clear assessments of intracranial hemorrhage. CT scans, on the other hand, are able to provide direct visualization of intracranial hemorrhage as well as where the hemorrhage is localized in the brain (i.e., subdural space, extradural space, etc.) (Rubin). Besides this, CT scans, among other types of imaging modalities, play a big role in assessing and visualizing injuries in many other tissues and organs of the body as well.

Notably, CT greatly aids in the identification of blunt abdominal trauma injuries. Prior to the use of CT in diagnostic abdominal imaging, techniques were insufficient in providing a comprehensive view of injuries to the peritoneum (lining of the abdominal cavity) — barium studies were unable to diagnose intra- and extraperitoneal abnormalities, while exploratory surgery was invasive and often lacked the ability to identify retroperitoneal abnormalities. CT is able to holistically image the peritoneum and the majority of other abdominal structures, thus making it easier for physicians to identify and locate injuries and treat them. Virtually all causes of abdominal pain, with the exception of acute cholecystitis, can be diagnosed using CT (Rubin). Additionally, CT scans have proved to be an excellent diagnostic tool for appendicitis, which is commonly misdiagnosed as there is a high rate of false negatives for this condition using traditional lab testing techniques. Not only does CT effectively minimize the incidence of these false negatives, but it also provides greater acuity and diagnostic accuracy than ultrasonography, another imaging technique commonly used for appendicitis. It is estimated that ultrasonography provides diagnostic accuracy rates of 71 to 97 percent, whereas CT provides much higher diagnostic accuracy rates between 93 to 98 percent (Old et al. 71). Other traumatic injuries that CT is frequently used to visualize and diagnose include injuries of the spleen, blunt aortic injury, skeletal pelvic and spinal injuries, renal colic, and many more (Rubin).

Overall, advancements in CT have been incredibly effective in diagnosing pathologies and general abnormalities, thereby rendering old diagnostic and imaging techniques obsolete. The use of CT in emergency departments has been shown to effectively reduce hospital admission rates, direct patient care, and decrease the average duration of patient hospital stays (Rubin).

Limitations and Overutilization of CT Scans

CT scanning technology, while greatly advanced, is still evolving constantly. While CT scanning technology has dramatically improved over the years and has become optimized in aiding the diagnosis of various pathologies, it still has not yet been optimized in aiding the diagnosis of others. Specific investigations into how to best use CT scans to diagnose and assess injuries/pathologies in a particular tissue or organ of the body are frequently being launched, ultimately progressing towards optimizing CT scanning techniques for their use in everyday medicine.

Still, shortcomings exist in everyday medicine with this type of technology. Exposure to ionizing radiation is a major topic of interest that is being investigated by countless researchers, as the long-term effects of this radiation are still largely not known. Other chapters in this book discuss concerns related to radiation levels in more detail.

While CT scans are undoubtedly a revolutionary technology, producing high resolution images to aid in the assessment of countless internal organs and structures, overutilization of CT scans in everyday medicine remains an issue. Not only is the overutilization of CT scans concerning due to the fact that it exposes patients to unnecessary radiation which can be harmful, but it also ignores patient welfare and the burdensome financial costs associated with this technology. Various factors influence overutilization of CT scans, which include (but are not limited to): self-referrals, defensive medicine, accidental requesting of inappropriate procedures, and duplicate imaging studies (Hendee et al. 241). Self-referral is defined as when a physician refers a patient for a procedure, in which that physician is also the service provider or the physician benefits financially by providing the service. In this case, a conflict of interest is deemed to be the motivating force at play, as the financial benefit that a physician reaps from the imaging procedure would seemingly override the question of whether the procedure is medically necessary or not. Self-referral is estimated to cost $16 billion per year for all unnecessary imaging procedures in the US (Hendee et al. 242). A seven-fold increase in medical radiation dose to the US population has also been observed in the last 25 years, which some experts also attribute to self-referral (Hendee et al. 242).

Defensive medicine, on the other hand, involves administering CT scans primarily to safeguard against possible accusations of malpractice (Hendee et al. 242). Rather than the principal motive being patient benefit, defensive medicine overestimates medical necessity and exposes the patient to unnecessary radiation in order to protect the hospital and the physician's own career from litigation. Another factor contributing to overutilization is the requesting of inappropriate procedures. Several physicians who request CT scans often have little knowledge about the technique itself, and the possibility of alternative tests/procedures that may yield similar or better results with a lower cost and less exposure to radiation. Another possibility is that physicians may have inadequate information about the patient or failed to be thorough in their examination, thus the physician may have requested an inappropriate imaging procedure. While such scenarios could be solved by radiologists actively screening every radiologic study requested by referring physicians in theory, this is much too unrealistic to expect (Hendee et al. 243).

Conclusion

Conclusively, this chapter has reviewed the specific applications of CT scans in everyday medicine by pinpointing and diagnosing abnormalities of nearly every part of the body. CT scans are specifically useful in efficiently assessing a patient's injuries when they have undergone trauma, as well as guiding treatment plans for cancer and other conditions. Evidently, the use of CT scans has become exceedingly widespread in modern medicine, with approximately 76 million CT scans performed in 2013 (Rubin). Over the years, CT scanning techniques have become optimized and specifically catered to visualize many different organs and tissues, yet the field is still growing and has enormous unrealized potential in managing many pathologies such as coronary heart disease and colon cancer. All in all, in spite of its overutilization and the dangers of its radiation, CT scanning has undoubtedly dramatically enhanced the health and survival of countless individuals worldwide.

CHAPTER 6

Basic Principles of CT Scans

Maggie Wang

Due to the prevalent use of CT scanning equipment in everyday medicine, understanding the fundamentals of how this piece of imaging equipment works is integral to optimizing its operation. CT scans are a form of X-ray imaging where cross-sectional images of an area of interest within a patient are generated. These images are then compiled using computerized algorithms to provide physicians with a 3-dimensional view of relevant structures, including significant structural landmarks and potential abnormalities/tumors. In the following chapter, the mechanics of CT machinery and the imaging process will be explored in depth.

CT Machinery

The CT imaging system is comprised of the gantry and the patient table, both of which work in conjunction to effectively capture the area of interest within the patient's body as a 3-dimensional image. The gantry is the ring-shaped component of the CT scanner, containing the majority of the machinery necessary to produce and detect X-rays. This machinery — the X-ray tube and detector — are closely linked together, working concurrently to sweep the X-ray beam through the patient's body and then detect the beam emerging on the other side. The patient table is what the patient lies on while being scanned, and this slowly moves through the gantry (Bell).

The X-ray tube is responsible for creating the X-ray, working to convert electrical energy that it receives into X-rays and heat. This electrical energy is fed by a generator, which creates an alternating current that is translated into a direct current when required, in order to ensure that there is a consistent and unidirectional flow of electrons travelling through the circuit. The tube consists of a filament and a target, which act as a cathode and anode, respectively. These components are both contained in an envelope that aids in providing vacuum, support and electrical insulation. This envelope is typically made from glass, but can also be composed of ceramic or metal. Through a process called thermionic emission, the filament is able to accelerate electrons using an extremely high voltage to ensure that they collide with the focal spot on the target. Once the electrons strike this target, they are able to produce X-rays as they are converted into photons. The radiation source created is a monochromatic X-ray beam that is composed of photons of the same wavelength. Within the tube, both the quality and quantity of X-rays can be controlled by adjusting parameters on the machinery. These factors are the kV, which is the tube voltage (i.e., the potential difference across the tube), mA, which is the tube current (i.e., flow through the tube) and the exposure time (Bell).

The X-ray beam is able to collimate at two points — one close to the X-ray tube and the other at the detector, where they fall into alignment. Focusing on the X-ray detector, there are two types of detectors that can be used. Scintillation detectors are more common and consist of a scintillation crystal and light detector. The scintillation crystal is able to fluoresce when struck by an x-photon and there is an attached device called a photodiode. The photodiode works to transform this light into electrical energy that can be collected by detector elements attached to a circuit board. Typical materials that are used for these detectors are cadmium tungstate, cesium iodide, bismuth germinate, etc. On the other hand, gas filled detectors work on the premise that a signal can be produced when the gas within the chamber is ionized by X-rays. Although scintillation detectors are more common, these gas filled detectors are cheaper, easier to calibrate and extremely stable. The most common type are xenon gas ionizable chambers, which contain a chamber filled with pressurized xenon gas. These contain three tungsten plates that work to ionize the photon that enters the channel, accelerate and amplify the ions between plates and then process the electric current and store it as digital data (Harmonay).

CT Scanning Mechanism

When the CT scanning machinery was first created, the founder envisioned the mechanism to be concurrent divisions of the subject into axial slices. This has since served to be the basis of CT scans, although various aspects of the process have changed with evolving technologies. Depending on the desired slice thickness, the X-ray beam used can be narrowed accordingly (Goldman, "Principles of CT and CT Technology"). In the case of scintillation detectors, the detector is then able to convert these X-rays into pulses of visible light to be stored by the computerized image reconstruction system. As the pulses of visible light correspond to the intensity of the X-ray, the energy of the photons that strike the detector can be quantified using proportionality calculations (Zezo).

Translation occurs when the X-ray tube and detector work with one another to scan the subject of interest. When each X-ray beam travels through the subject of interest and hits the detector to be stored as digital data, each individual beam is termed and quantified as a ray. As multiple beams travel through the subject during a translation, the collection of all the X-rays are known as a view. In order to obtain a more complete scan, the

X-ray tube and detector simultaneously rotate approximately 1 degree where another view is translated. Nowadays, most scanners are able to collect over 750 rays/view and the translation process is repeated 1000+ times over 360 degrees. This entire process is called translate-rotate motion, which serves as the foundations of first generation CT geometry. In essence, linear translation occurs to produce a view, which is then followed by rotation in small increments and the process is repeated until a complete 3-dimensional depiction is generated (Goldman, "Principles of CT and CT Technology").

Fundamentals of CT Imaging

The translate-rotate mechanism is then translated into CT imagery, as cross-sectional slices of the patient form a matrix. The matrix is composed of 3-dimensional boxes of subject tissue that are termed voxels. Depending on the scan circle (i.e., the circular area that the X-ray measurements were obtained over) as well as the size of the matrix (i.e., rows and columns that split the scan circle), the x and y dimensions of the voxel are determined. These dimensions lie on the plane of the slice and are often just referred to as pixel size. The z dimension on the other hand, is dependent on the thickness of the slice in question. Overall, the construction of the CT image in this matrix format is utilized to determine the level of attenuation the X-ray beam measures within each voxel (Goldman, "Principles of CT and CT Technology").

When ionizing radiation is transmitted through an object of some form, properties of the object can be translated into an image based on the X-ray absorption on the detector. This absorption is quantified as what's known as the linear attenuation coefficient (μ) and is reflective of the degree that a material is able to reduce X-ray intensity. This value is dependent on distinct properties of the tissue, including atomic number and density of the material. Computerized systems are able to transform these linear attenuation coefficient measurements into CT numbers that are quantified on a scale called the Hounsfield unit (HU) scale. This is done by calculating a relationship between the linear attenuation coefficient of the material measured and water using the following equation: CTtissue= (μtissue- μwater)μwater1000. The Hounsfield unit scale describes radiodensity and has significant implications on a physician's ability to compare tissue composition and detect abnormalities. When applied in CT imaging, a CT number of -1000 is indicative of a voxel containing air whereas a number of 1000 indicates a voxel containing dense, cortical bone. A number of 0 would indicate a voxel containing water. Utilizing this quantification system, tissue composition directly corresponds to CT number range. For instance, the lungs have a CT number range of -830 to -200, fat has a range of -250 to -30 and blood has a range of 20-80. These values are approximations however, and vary depending on the CT acquisition method as filters, reconstruction algorithms, etc., may slightly alter the values (Goldman, "Principles of CT and CT Technology").

The quantization of attenuation into CT numbers poses a problem when the matrix is applied to a computer display, however. The CT image is displayed on a monitor for immediate viewing by physicians, which typically have a display matrix of 512x512 pixels. However, displays only have approximately 256 shades of gray. Thus, the full CT number range of -1000 to +1000 must be distributed amongst only 256 discernable levels of gray. This limits the ability of the physician to distinguish between some soft-tissue structures. Despite the CT numbers between a structure and its surroundings differing, they could be invisible as they fall within the same range that is encompassed in a single gray level. In order to resolve this problem, a technique called windowing has been employed, which provides CT viewers with the ability to decide how CT numbers are allocated to gray levels. Viewers are able to specify both a window width and length. The length serves as the center CT number, whereas the width provides a range of CT numbers both above and below the center. These values are formatted as (W:x L:y) in Hounsfield units on a computer. When applying this windowing method, physicians tend to follow a guide that indicates the (W:x L:y) that pertains to varying sections of the body. When a CT scan is being taken of the head and neck, a physician that is interested in viewing the subdural region would likely select a window of (W:130-300 L:50-100). To image the liver in the abdomen, a physician would likely select a window of (W:1500 L:-600) (Zezo).

CT Image Quality

The image quality of CT scans are dependent on four factors: contrast resolution, spatial resolution, image noise and artifacts. These aspects of CT imaging interplay to establish sensitivity, which is the visibility of details as well as the viewer's ability to detect low contrast structures. Through understanding this, those who work with CT imaging are able to play around with different forms of CT machinery and the settings in order to determine the best means of ensuring that the structure of interest is visible (i.e., fatty tumors, bone abnormalities, etc.). In addition, more knowledge allows for the balance between radiation dose and image quality to be optimized, as increased radiation dose tends to enhance the factors that improve sensitivity yet raises concerns about patient safety (Goldman, "Principles of CT: Radiation Dose and Image Quality").

Contrast Resolution

CT contrast resolution is the ability to distinguish between varying intensities on the digital image. Both subject contrast and display contrast factor into this, but subject contrast is the main variable of interest as a result of the arbitrary nature of display contrast (dependent on windowing settings). Subject contrast is largely determined by differential attenuation, which as described previously, is the difference in X-ray attenuation. In other words, this variable represents the differences in X-ray intensity that the detector then translates into voxel detailing (Goldman, "Principles of CT: Radiation Dose and Image Quality"). The contrast resolution of CT scans fails to be intrinsically high, due to the X-ray attenuation differential usually being small between various tissues. However, factors that contribute to contrast resolution can be altered in order to optimize viewing abilities. A study by Lin and Alessio explored the contrast resolution of cardiac CT scans and concluded that the most effective means of increasing contrast resolution was through external means rather than directly altering the machinery. By administering intravenous iodinated contrast, contrast resolution between structures with a high level of administered contrast and their surroundings was relatively high. Furthermore, by altering the timing, increasing iodine flux and maintaining contrast volume, this mechanism further enhances contrast resolution. The authors also determined that decreasing X-ray tube voltage was effective in increasing the contrast resolution of cardiac CTs, as the photoelectric effect promotes opacification of blood vessels and increases visibility. However, altering CT machinery settings proves to be controversial, as not only does decreasing tube voltage simultaneously increase image noise, but it also raises concerns involving the radiation dose administered to the individual during the scan. Thus, contrast material proves to be the best means of increasing contrast resolution and the study serves as a reminder of the importance to maintain a balance between quality and safety when working with X-rays (Lin and Alessio).

Spatial Resolution

CT spatial resolution is another factor that plays into the quality of CT imaging and is defined as the ability to distinguish small, closely spaced objects on an image. The X-ray detector plays a large role in determining this; in particular, this factor is dependent on the size of the detector measurements and the spacing of the detector measurements that are used to reconstruct the image (aperture). In particular, a small aperture and closely spaced measurements are preferred. Additionally, excessively large display pixels and image reconstruction processes may also contribute to spatial resolution. As the image is first reconstructed using matrix pixels that are called voxels and then translated onto the display screen, issues with resolution arise when the display pixels are larger than those of the reconstruction matrix. In order to resolve this issue, the majority of modern scanners have graphic zoom features. In terms of image reconstruction, computerized softwares apply reconstruction filters during filtered backprojection resolution. The best filter should be the ideal compromise between spatial resolution and image noise. Removing the majority of the image blur would result in too sharp of a CT scan that is corrupted by image noise and appears grainy. Thus, filters are selected to ensure that there is still some blur to reduce image noise and produce improved diagnostic quality and spatial resolution (Goldman, "Principles of CT: Radiation Dose and Image Quality").

Image Noise

CT image noise is a result of random fluctuations in CT numbers of uniform materials that are detected by the machinery, which manifest as grainy appearances on the reconstructed image. This aspect of CT imagery is largely influenced by the numbers of photons in the X-ray beams that are processed within each section of the image; however, rather than being a result of complications with the individual pixels, the detector measurements have the largest impact. In order to combat the graininess of the image, there are various factors that can alter the X-ray beam, thus changing the number of photons that are able to strike the detector. The X-ray tube amperage allows for changes to be made in beam intensity as the mA value is altered, which in turn changes the number of X-rays produced. If the X-ray beam width is altered (i.e., the thickness of each slice), then the number of X-rays also changes proportionally. For example, increasing the width from 2 mm to 4 mm would double the number of X-rays that are recognized by the detector. Finally, increasing the peak kilovoltage would also increase the levels of X-rays that are able to penetrate the patient to be processed by the detector. Apart from alterations that are made to the CT machinery itself in order to reduce image noise, reconstruction filters also play a role. As mentioned previously, smooth filters are able to blur image noise and thus reduce the visual impact. These filters tend to be preferred in soft tissues as noise has more interference than blur does. Conversely, sharp filters help to enhance image noise and are preferred in tissues such as bone, where blur is more interfering than noise (Goldman, "Principles of CT: Radiation Dose and Image Quality").

Image Artifacts

Image artifacts are the final factor that play a role in altering quality of CT images. In essence, artifacts are structures that although seen on the image produced, are not reflective of the actual anatomy of the patient. These artifacts fall into three categories: shading artifacts, ring artifacts and streak artifacts (Goldman, "Principles of CT: Radiation Dose and Image Quality").

The most common form of shading artifacts are beam-hardening effects, which are non-uniformities in CT numbers of a uniform material and are a result of problems with beam-hardening corrections. Although these artifacts are present on all CT images to some extent and typically are not apparent unless a narrow windowing setting is used, they can obscure visibility when the scan passes through thicker regions of bone or contrast mediums. When this occurs, increased amounts of hardening occur, which results in regions of hypointensity (CT numbers that are too low) appearing downstream the paths of the rays (Goldman, "Principles of CT: Radiation Dose and Image Quality").

Ring artifacts are a result of issues with measurement inaccuracies of a detector as compared to those of its neighbours in the array. This includes errors, imbalances, calibration drifts, etc. These are typically associated with third generation scan geometry, as these detectors measure the X-ray at a distance d from the center of rotation. As d is dependent on where the detector is within the overall array, problems with measurements that are associated with a single detector could be backprojected along additional rays that are measured by that same detector. Although this only slightly affects the pixels, they can reinforce an ring-like artifact with a radius of d. Improvements in software ring-correction algorithms are usually highly effective in detecting and fixing these ring formations (Goldman, "Principles of CT: Radiation Dose and Image Quality").

Streak artifacts are commonly due to problematic detector measurements that are a result of either motion (i.e., movement results in the same anatomy appearing in different locations), insufficient intensity in the X-ray beam or malfunctions in the detector. However, software algorithms are again able to detect these issues and correct them. In order to avoid streak artifacts, many CT scanning systems perform a process called overscanning, where the X-ray beam and detector scan past 360 degrees to reduce any streaks that may be a result of motion (Goldman, "Principles of CT: Radiation Dose and Image Quality").

Conclusion

In any context, the ability to understand the fundamentals of a process is crucial to make improvements and enhance application within real world settings. This chapter delved into the fundamentals and the interplay between various aspects of CT scans, including the machinery, the translate-rotate process, image reconstruction and quality-altering improvements. These principles can then be drawn upon to optimize the function and operation of CT scans in everyday medicine, which have substantial implications on patient diagnosis and medical understanding.

CHAPTER 7

What is still unknown?

Alexander Martin

The CT Scan has become progressively popular in modern medical practices since the 1980s. CT scans have changed the way medicine is universally practiced. Here, CT scans enable physicians the ability to investigate the body through the device's multiple X-rays. The medical field has benefited tremendously because of their use. Cancers can be detected early, for instance. However, there is still a lot of conflicting information regarding the benefits of its use. Specifically, whether CT scans are harmful or not. There is still a lot of information regarding CT scans that is still not known. Specifically, if their use could promote various cancers in the body through the radiation received from the treatment. This narrative can be analyzed to see why people believe this and if there is any truth to it. Factors such as overprescription of CT scans could be a leading cause if it were the case. Ideas including this will be highlighted in the following chapter: the topic will be explored, and prominent studies will be contrasted to reveal what is currently known.

Is Ionized Radiation Associated with Cancer?

The main unknown surrounding CT scans are whether they cause cancer. Analyzing this idea, CT scans take images of the whole body which exposes a patient to high levels of radiation. During this process one receives ionizing radiation, which penetrates the tissue, organs, and bones of the body. Ionizing radiation is defined as "high-energy radiation that has enough energy to remove an electron (negative particle) from an atom or molecule, causing it to become ionized" (National Cancer Institute). Everyday people are exposed to ionized radiation daily. For example, the sun emits natural radiation. However, when patients are exposed to high levels of ionizing radiation, they can deplete their cells' natural ability to heal (Burgio et al). Similar to the sun, if ionized radiation is controlled, individuals are less exposed to risk. It is known that "Children are at a greater risk than adults of developing cancer after being exposed to ionizing radiation" (Kutanzi et al). The events which took place in both Hiroshima and Nagasaki in Japan, during World War 2, serves as an analogy to discuss this concept. Two atomic bombs "Fat Man" and "Little Boy" were dropped on the populations of the two cities. As a result, Japanese people were exposed to high levels of ionizing radiation. After the fact, the cancer leukemia was found in atomic bomb survivors who were exposed to these high levels of radiation from the explosions. Here, there was a significant increase in cases of Leukemia 3 years after initial exposure (Ibid). Also, "Analysis in the Life Span Study of Japanese atomic bomb survivors indicated [there were] 310 deaths due to leukemia during the period of 1950-2000 in 866,111 people" (Ibid). There is significant information that suggests that children exposed to ionized radiation levels could be more likely to develop cancers, such as leukemia. However, there is a limitation in this study; it does not discuss how much or for how long everyone was initially exposed to the ionizing radiation. Thus, it is unclear whether modern use of CT scans can pose the same risks. CT scans use ionized radiation to complete their X-rays. It is noted that, "the effects [of] prolonged exposure to low doses... are the most frequent and most dangerous for human [beings]" (Burgio et al). What is still unclear is whether low exposure to it results in the same effects. Notably, studies fail to provide a full picture of the situation. Studies use blatant language that indicates whether CT scans are the direct issue. Therefore, it makes it hard to determine whether CT scans cause cancer or if genetics is a main factor for the various cancer cases. Understanding what information and studies are important when trying to reveal the truth of the matter.

Possible Overprescription of CT Scans

People are being prescribed CT scans more than is required. There are multiple medical practices that do not require radiation and are just as effective as a CT scan. For example, magnetic resonance imaging (MRI) and ultrasounds are known to be much safer than CT scans because of this (Redberg and Smith-Bindman). Both methods are known to not cause cancer and are possible alternatives considering it is still generally unknown. Currently, "One in 10 Americans undergo a CT scan every year, and many of them get more than one" (Ibid). Also, dosage and levels of radiation depending on the institution administering them fluctuate. Depending on the physician's opinion, "the dose at one hospital can be as much as 50 times stronger than at another" (Ibid). Keeping this in mind, CT scans are possibly overprescribed considering the risk potential; studies are still debating its long-term effects. Susan G Komen of the Institute of Medicine noted "radiation from medical imaging, and hormone therapy, the use of which has substantially declined in the last decade, were the leading environmental causes of breast cancer, and advised that women reduce their exposure to unnecessary CT scans" (Ibid). Here, breast cancer was found in women who received excessive CT scans. Possibly this is incidental, but it should still be considered regarding the debate. Measures are being put in place to address this issue and find a clear answer. For example, the topic is progressively being addressed in medical journals where physicians can better understand the risks associated with the treatment. The American College of Radiology and the American College of Cardiology provided appropriateness criteria for the potential that CT scans cause cancers. Here, "The guidelines are developed and reviewed annually by expert panels in diagnostic imaging and interventional radiology. Each panel includes leaders in radiology and other specialties" (American College of Radiology). Evidently, there is progress being made to answer the question for certain. There are now radiology benefit managers who assess a specific patients' situation and determine whether the test is absolutely necessary, for instance (Redberg and Smith-Bindman). Thus, there is a narrative being formed around the idea that CT scans tests are overused and overprescribed. There continues to be a lot of conflicting information regarding the truth. Further studies continue to reveal this. Going forward, it is important to recognize that there is a lot of uncertainty concerning the topic that CT scans cause cancer. However, safety measures are progressively finding their way to the medical field. Overall, it should be considered that CT scans are possibly being overprescribed given the uncertainty of its potential to cause various cancers.

Conflicting Information

There is a lot of conflicting information regarding whether CT scans lead to future cancer cases. Understanding what information and studies are available should be considered to determine the possible truth. To start, it is helpful to investigate the treatments and processes more indepthly to reflect on the device's potentiality of causing cancer. Briefly discussed prior, CT scan consists of a radiograph that takes multiple X-rays of an individual piece or multiple parts of the body. These scans are projected through the body and recorded onto a sheet of film where a physician can analyze it. Here, a 3D object of the body is converted to a 2D object through the process which requires radiation. Significantly, different body parts require different levels of radiation. Bone is a lot denser and requires more radiation than the lungs, for instance. People are becoming concerned about excessive exposure to radiation. Notably, "over 80 million CT scans are performed in the United States each year, compared [to] just three million in 1980 (Harvard Medical School)." The popularization of the practice has created debate about whether exposure to the radiation of CT scans is harmful or not. This idea came to fruition after two physicians named Rita Redberg and Rebecca Smith-Binman came out about their concern that CT scans may inevitably lead to cancer. The two took their opinion to The New York Times and published the article "We are giving ourselves cancer" in 2014. Here, it highlights the idea that modern medical practices are "...irradiating ourselves to death" (Redberg and Smith-Bindman). Currently not much is known about the effects of the radiation on the body from CT scans, but excessive exposure to radiation continues to be at an all-time high. Consider that, "The radiation doses of CT scans (a series of X-ray images from multiple angles) are 100 to 1,000 times higher than conventional X-rays)" (Ibid). The article continues to focus on the fact that there is sufficient epidemiologic evidence that supports the notion that CT causes cancer. It notes that "A single CT scan exposes a patient to the amount of radiation that... shows can be cancer causing" (Ibid). The article's claims should be considered, but there are still conflicting opinions. For instance, the Mayo Clinic believes that CT scans pros outway the cons. The Mayo Clinic claims that CT scans in fact do not have significant levels of ionized radiation, especially that could cause cancer. Their article, "Answers to Common Questions About the Use and Safety of CT Scans," notes that "...at the low dose associated with a CT scan the risk either is too low to be convincingly demonstrated or does not exist..." to cause cancer. The Mayo Clinic discusses this further throughout their article "Answers to Common Questions About the Use and Safety of CT Scans" (Mayo Clinic). Here, it discusses physicians' use of a calculated effective dose when considering patients' radiation levels for their CT scans. An effective dose is based on the known levels that cause radiation, which is measured in millisieverts (mSv). Considering this, "CT Scans range from less than 1 to approximately 10 mSv. Compare this to the fact that individuals exposed to environmental radiation such as the sun receive only 3 mSv (Mayo Clinic). It is uncertain whether the max increase of 7mSv could result in possible cancer. Again, different parts of the body require different levels of radiation to deliver an effective X-ray. Radiation "...exposure from a body CT scan is approximately 1 to 2 mSv whereas the exposure from a body CT scan is approximately 10 mSv. However, when multiple CT scans are done at once it could promote damage. An individual in a scenario like this could receive up to 20 to 30 mSv in a single session (Mayo Clinic). There are findings Found that people exposed to 200 mSv began to develop leukemia two years after their initial exposure. Again, it is unclear whether a certain low exposure could trigger the same results. Lastly, not much is known about the effects of radiation levels of CT scans on the body, and if they cause cancer or not. Radiation levels should always be as low as possible as a precautionary, given the conflicting information. Overall, more direct studies are needed to clarify the issue for the public. Right now, there is still limited information available on whether it is, so everything at this point is speculative.

In-Conclusive Studies

Radiation levels should be the main concern of physicians. The study "Computed tomography - an increasing source of radiation exposure" also found that CT scans cause cancer. However, this study is highly controversial and uses a cancer-risk model from another study by the National Academies of Science. The study is controversial because it concluded that there is limited data to suggest that ionizing radiation promotes cancer growth in individuals due to direct instances. Reviewing the study, the article's conclusions are tainted by the fact that there is no sufficient evidence to base their claims. Therefore, the study's findings should be ill considered as a result.

Again, this is another incidence that conveys that the truth is still unclear whether CT scans in fact cause cancer growth. Since it is unknown, radiation levels should be prioritized on being as low as possible as a safety precaution. CT scans pose a double-edged sword; Possible cancers can be revealed through its use, but its use can also potentially promote various cancers. Notably, "CT alone contributes to almost one half of the total radiation exposure from medical use and one quarter of the average radiation exposure per capita in the USA" (Yu et al). It is becoming more routine to control the radiation levels because of the concern that high levels of ionized radiation cause cancer, as discussed prior. The BMJ published by the trade union of the British Medical Association which focused on people's exposure to ionized radiation specifically. Their article, "Cancer risk in 680,000 people exposed to computed tomography scans in childhood or adolescence: data linkage study of 11 million Australians," found a correlation between CT scans and cancer rates (Matthews et al). In synopsis, the study noted that there were 60,7474 cancers incidences in people exposed to a CT scan at least one year before a diagnosis. The study's results found those who received excessive exposure to ionized radiation were 24% more likely to develop cancer in their lifetime (Matthews et al). The conclusion of the findings noted that there could be a connection, but again, it is still uncertain whether CT radiation has a direct connection to cancer (Ibid). The test-subjects had an average of 9.5 years from their initial exposure to the ionized radiation. There is a debate whether the cancers recorded were genetic or the result of their CT scans. Again, there is limited statistics about the matter which makes it hard to compare the findings. Also, there are flaws in the conduction of the BMJ study. The findings were based around individuals who are aged 0-19. Here, the statistics are not associated with people later in their lifetimes. This feeds into the narrative that the test-subjects' cancers could possibly be genetic. Overall, the findings were conflicting and inclusive as a result. Again, it is unclear whether CT directly causes cancer or whether genetics plays a main role.

Conclusion

There is a lot that is still unknown about CT scans. The popularization and effects of its use should not go unquestioned. Although there are no direct studies that answer this question, precautions can be taken to ensure one's safety in the process. For instance, if one is regularly exposed, discussing the concern that CT scans cause cancer with a physician could be the first step. There are alternative treatments that could be taken to limit radiation exposure. MRIs and ultrasounds are other popular treatments that can be just as effective as CT scans. Also, they do not use ionizing radiation in their processes and are not harmful. Being conscious about what is unknown about the potential dangers of CT scans is important. People need to weigh the pros and cons with a knowledgeable physician on the matter. However, CT scans should not be disregarded because of these speculations. CT scans are still an effective treatment that helps doctors reveal possible cancers; it saves lives and is a significant medical breakthrough when trying to understand the human body. There is more to be done to ensure that people are safe from the potential harms of the process. Being conscious of this, individuals should understand the effects of radiation levels, over-exposure, and the risks. Overall, there is a lot that is still uncertain about CT scans. More studies are needed to answer the question of whether overexposure contributes to various cancers.

CHAPTER 8

Use of CT in children

Tenzin Yehshopa

CT (computed tomography) is a non-invasive procedure and as mentioned in previous chapters, can execute cross-sectional images of human bodies. These scans can provide more information and detailed imaging of children's bones, tissues, and blood vessels than conventional X-rays and often is the first choice of modelling during emergencies since it offers rapid results (Boston Children's Hospital). Imaging studies that use ionizing radiation are an essential tool for the evaluation of many disorders of childhood. However, there is still some ongoing debate regarding whether or not it's harmful to use CT scans on children. Various studies out there suggest that radiation used in the tests increases children's lifelong risk of cancer. The key ideas covered in this chapter is examining the possible risks associated with the use of CT in children and what experts are trying to do to combat and minimize these risks.

CT Procedure for Children

In children, CT is often used to investigate injuries to the head, or other neurological issues in relation to hearing loss, fractures and breathing issues. The use of CT in children is an excellent way to find the root of the problem in an efficient way minimizing the cost of time. One may request a CT scan to obtain specific diagnostic information which can be complementary to other imaging technologies used in a hospital setting. Other imaging technologies can include X-ray, ultrasound, nuclear medicine or for an MRI (Goske). For children, CT scanning can be life saving as it will quickly reveal internal injuries and bleeding and provide important information to the medical team. Since CT scans are generally quick, often averaging less than 10 seconds, many children can hold still for the entire procedure (Boston Children's Hospital). But depending on which part of the body is being scanned, the exam can be a longer process. Some of these scans are more forgiving of slight movements, while others require the child to be entirely motionless for a greater length of time. Depending on the child's age and other factors, anesthesia may be necessary. CT scans can be performed on newborns, infants and older children including teens (Cooks Children's). In children CT is typically used to diagnose causes of abdominal pain and evaluate for injury after trauma (Pearce et al). Other common uses is to diagnose cancer, monitor response to treatment for cancer, and diagnose and monitor infectious or inflammatory disorders (Pearce et al). CT may also be performed to evaluate blood vessels throughout the body. With CT, it is possible to obtain very detailed pictures of the heart and blood vessels in children, even newborn infants. Other than a chest X-ray, CT is the most commonly used imaging procedure for evaluating the chest (Boston Children's Hospital). The use of CT in children can be used to evaluate complications from infections such as pneumonia, a tumor that arises in the lung or has spread there from a distant site, airway disease such as inflammation of the bronchi, birth defects, trauma to blood vessels or lungs (Radiology Info). CT is well-suited for visualizing diseases or injury of important organs in the abdomen including the liver, kidney and spleen. However, there are risks to CT scans which will be examined in the next portion of this chapter.

Potential Risks

It has long been recognized that individuals who are exposed to high doses of ionizing radiation are known to be at risk of developing cancer in their lifetime. CT scans involve ionizing radiation as is used in conventional X-rays (Bulas). It is important to understand for the overall purpose of discussion that radiation is an essential component of CT examination and the cause and effect relationship between CT examinations and development of cancer has no direct link, so they must be estimated. In certain clinical situations, the benefits of an accurate diagnosis outweigh the risk of exposure to radiation during the exam. Despite this information, there is no conclusive evidence that radiation from diagnostic X-rays causes cancer. However, some studies of large populations exposed to radiation have demonstrated slight increases in cancer risk even at low levels of radiation exposure, particularly in children (Goske). To be safe, and for the sake of children who need CT scans, it is important to keep in mind that low doses of radiation may cause harm. The risk for radiation induced cancers in children should be evaluated against the statistical risk of developing cancer in the entire population (Brenner et al). Statements that are based on expert panel reviews of available information are additional sources of estimates of the risks of low-level radiation. The BEIR Committee of the National Academy of Sciences in the past few years concluded that the "risk of cancer proceeds in a linear fashion at lower doses without a threshold and that the smallest dose has the potential to cause a small increased risk to humans" (National Research Council). The overall risk of a cancer death over a person's lifetime is estimated to be 20-25% (New York State Department of Health). The estimated increased risk of cancer over a person's lifetime from a single CT scan is controversial but has been estimated to be a fraction of this risk of only 0.03- 0.05% (New York State Department of Health). These estimates for the population as a whole do not represent a direct risk to one child. This information merely shows that the risk of developing cancer related to a single CT scan is very small, but the available research indicates that there may be some risk and the risk may be cumulative. Experts calibrate X-ray-based equipment and adapt protocols to deliver doses appropriate to children (Radiology Info). The narrow beams of radiation used in CT, as well as protective shielding that prevents unnecessary radiation to sensitive tissues, also help limit radiation dose (Boston Children's Hospital). For children, the most common scenario is that of head injury. In past years many pediatricians have played it safe and ordered head scans for minor head injuries that were very unlikely to have such serious consequences. They go down this route in order to look for signs of a fracture or of bleeding around the brain that would be life-threatening if undetected and untreated. Sometimes, it is possible to reach a diagnosis by using imaging technologies that do not involve radiation. Some examples include ultrasound or magnetic resonance imaging (MRI). When appropriate, the radiologists will advise referring physicians that this could potentially be the safest course of action to take.

There are other external risks in relation to CT scans in children. Leaking fluid at the IV site ruptures as well as allergic reaction to iodinated contrast material can also be an issue which is common in children who are allergic to iodine or shellfish (Bulas et al). These allergic reactions can be due to contrasting dyes used depending on the CT scan, most commonly used for abdominal CT scans in children (Bulas et al). There is also a potential risk of kidney damage from IV contrast dye. Although rare, it is most likely to occur for children with pre-existing kidney problems (Boston Children's Hospital). Some children also may experience hives, itching or wheezing as a result. Although these reactions are rare and not usually serious, it does pose a health risk that patients and parents should be notified of. Exacerbation of renal failure in children with preexisting renal disease is also a risk that needs to be considered. In children, the allergic reaction risk using nonionic contrast is thankfully quite low. However, for younger children or others who cannot cooperate, sedation adds a risk to CT as well (Bulas et al). During these procedures consent must be obtained before sedation or anesthesia for any reason. This is because some younger children who may not be able to hold still during a CT scan may need a brief period of anesthesia or sedation. Unfortunately in some children, this can cause headaches, shivering and vomiting (Bulas et al). The other risks such as allergies to iodine and renal function are carefully considered before the examination in most radiology departments (Bulas et al). If these risks are not examined it can lead to complications later on. One risk that is not typically discussed is the possible radiation risk from low-level ionizing radiation (Bulas et al). This lack of discussion occurs for several reasons. The first being that there is a lack of consensus among medical and scientific experts about the actual radiation risk from low-level radiation (Goske). Another reason why there is this issue is because there is a lack of awareness on the part of referring physicians as to possible risks. Due to this misinformation, community standards may not be discussing radiation as a potential risk. There is also research that emphasizes how conveying this complex topic to parents and caregivers in a straightforward format is extremely difficult (New York State Department of Health). Each of these reasons potentially hinders the discussion about the risk of CT.

Risk Mitigation

Most radiologists now accept the cancer risks are real, though very small. However, because of the great value of CT scans as a diagnostic tool, it would not be rational or feasible to abandon CT technology because of the risks. Nevertheless, the wide variations in CT use from country to country and from place to place indicates there is some overuse of CTs without corresponding clinical benefit. In addition to the powerful multidetector scanners used in hospital settings to minimize exam time they also often eliminate the need to sedate children. Since CT technology uses ionizing radiation, the equipment often used and the protocols made will be done in order to keep the doses "child-sized" and appropriate for their body proportions (Robbins). It is important that doses are as low as possible without compromising the image quality needed to make a correct diagnosis. One common way to reduce the radiation being exposed to children is to perform only the necessary CT examinations and to adjust the exposure levels for pediatric CT based on child size, region scanned and organ body scanned. It is important to stress that the absolute cancer risks associated with CT scans are small. A study last year found that children who had a CT before age 22 had a slightly higher risk of leukemia and brain tumors (Pearce et al). Physicians and medical professionals do have alternatives that they could use and implement during medical procedures. It would be useful if these options are presented to the child's primary caregiver so that they know their options and the risks associated. In some instances research has shown that Ultrasound machines and MRI scanners can be as good as CT in detecting appendicitis in children (Bajoghli et al). Neither of those alternatives use X-ray radiation, the kind that can damage genetic material. The most common CT scan in children is a head scan, given after a blow to the head. A CT scan would be ordered if it is likely that the child has a skull fracture or bleeding. Examination would be properly done if the child has signs of skull fracture, such as black eyes and bleeding (Cook Children's). Recent research indicates that most of the excess cancers in children and young age groups occurring more than two years after exposure have been caused by the radiation (Pearce et al). To reduce future risks, guidelines have been developed to allow minor head injuries to be managed by observation, and without the need for a CT scan. The overall professional response and new discussions around this issue has been to question the need for a CT scan for each child case. There is a prominent movement to make the radiation dose as low as can be achieved while still giving a good diagnostic image for children. People can start to consult guidelines endorsed by professional bodies and governments, by asking professionals whether the CT scan is really needed for their child, and whether there might be an available alternative diagnostic test (Pearce et al). Current approaches, involving patients and families, professional and regulatory bodies are helping to achieve a better balance between the risks and benefits of CT scanning as they are currently understood (Brenner et al). Over time, new research evidence will support improved guidelines that can better optimise the balance of risks and benefits for each and every patient. It is important to keep in mind that children are more radiosensitive than adults, this is why these mitigation techniques are important practices (Bajoghli). They also have a longer life expectancy over which they may develop cancer from exposures to ionizing radiation (Pearce et al).

The paediatric radiology and medical community has long had an awareness of this issue and has developed radiation protection policies and practices that reflect this (World Health Organization). With the increased use of imaging and in particular, CT scanning, there is increasing attention to this issue by the entire medical and radiology communities. Educational resources for health care providers as well as patients and parents have surged over the past decade. There are even collaborations done by several radiology, medical physics, paediatrics, and governmental organizations to increase awareness of radiation safety issues in children and to provide education to all stakeholders caring for children on ways to decrease the ionizing radiation exposure in children (World Health Organization). For parents, basic information brochures that can be printed or downloaded that describe what an X-ray is, what are its risks and benefits, and what can be done to decrease these risks. A call to action has been published advocating a reduction of ionizing radiation exposure to children by delivering the right imaging exam, the right way with the right dose. In June 2009, the World Health Organization (WHO) conducted a conference on children's health and environment in South Korea (World Health Organization). They suggested the principles of "safe use of radiation in pediatrics". Although there is progress towards more research and awareness of using radiation in pediatrics there are also ways to ensure children are not being exposed to radiation on a day to day basis.

Conclusion

Concerns about CT scans are understandable and questions should be encouraged, particularly when scientists are still discussing its impact on children. As mentioned in this chapter, imaging should be done when there is a clear medical benefit. The use of low amounts of radiation for adequate imaging based on the size of the child should be of the utmost importance. Imaging only the indicated areas will also decrease radiation exposure. Pediatricians can also suggest the use of alternative diagnostic studies such as ultrasound or MRI when possible and appropriate to do so. Although discussion of the relative risks of CT for children is complex and challenging in itself, it is important that information for pediatricians, parents and patients will help alleviate the confusion and promote the study of these potential areas of concern. It is the responsibility of those health care professionals who use CT scanning to ensure that each CT scan is required. It is also the responsibility of the radiology personnel to ensure that radiation risk is minimized by using strict protocols and principles to determine the correct techniques are being used. In summary, there is wide agreement that the benefits of an indicated CT scan far outweigh the risks.

CHAPTER 9

What does the general public think about X-rays?

Hannah Schepian

X ray scans have a lot to offer in the medical world, enabling medical health professionals to provide a more accurate diagnosis or treatment plan than without them. Although they have revolutionized the medical field, the general public do not always see eye to eye in terms of awareness and perception of these medical imaging tests, with healthcare professionals or even sometimes each other. Many lack the needed awareness to understand how x-rays work and their risks versus benefits and have sifted through so much misinformation over time from media, the internet, and those around them that they could have formed any perception of the subject. This is harmful as when the general public is not well informed, they risk making health care decisions that potentially lead to more harm than good. Overall physicians need to be aware of this when communicating an x-ray test to a patient and differentiate their language based on the needs of their patient.

With the constant advancement in medical imaging through history, alongside a vast spread of inconsistent and at times incorrect information, the knowledge of the general public surrounding x rays varies immensely (Freudenberg and Beyer). Whether patients receive insufficient information from medical professionals, inaccurate information from non-medical professionals, or rely on media, news or the internet to educate themselves on the subject, the general public's knowledge of radiation generally does not match current scientific opinion (Krewski et al. 629). To elaborate, discrepancies in public knowledge surrounding medical imaging mainly surround the understanding of radiation dose, as well as potential health risks linked to the imaging. In terms of the dose of radiation, Nuclear Medicine Communications conducted a survey aiming to evaluate patient's awareness about the levels of radiation they are being exposed to. The results evidenced that out of the 100 participants, with 38% reporting having some knowledge of radiation doses in nuclear medicine, "a low number of correct answers alongside a high number of 'I don't know' answers (Ribeiro et al. 586)." That being said, although over a third of participants claimed to be educated more or less on radiation doses, many were unable to correctly answer questions embodying radiation exposure. On the other hand, in regard to the general public's knowledge dealing with the subject of the potential health risks brought on by medical imaging such as x rays also did not correlate with current scientific research. A study of over 600 participants concluded that "few patients indicated that they had been made aware of any potential risks associated with x rays and other medical imaging tests by their medical health providers, with some of them pointing out that the only information received was in regard to how they should physically prepare for the test" (Lumbreras et al.). With that in mind, a significant number of individuals are either fully trusting their doctors to provide them with the optimal care, or they are deciding to rely on an alternative source for information about potential risks they could be subjected to. Overall, a great deal of the general public doesn't have adequate accurate information in association with the level of radiation exposure, as well as the accompanying risks of X-ray tests, let alone the scientific terms often used to understand explanations that are given by medical professionals.

While the lack of information that is provided by healthcare professionals contributes significantly to a patient's lack of awareness surrounding medical imaging, many other factors can potentially facilitate the procurement of misinformation surrounding the topic. While the varying spectrum of information easily accessible through the internet or media can offer fast answers and enhance the general public's awareness, people are often unequipped to separate what is factual or what is false. That being said, many people are self-educating, forming expectations, and making medical decisions based on partial and potentially incorrect information. It is made evident in the Journal of Nuclear Medicine Technology, that "between the testimonials of friends and family who have been x rayed, articles in magazines and newspapers, demonstrators and showmen, and all the other occult avenues through which information about the rays might be passed, a patient might have formed almost any impression" (Baldwin and Grantham 243). Taking that into consideration, individuals are at risk at making sense of the perceptions of non-medical professionals corresponding to medical image testing as facts and using them to make healthcare decisions of a nature that can potentially affect their diagnosis and treatment outcomes.

Hence, it is crucial that patients have a sufficient level of awareness surrounding X-rays and medical imaging, notably about the level of exposure to radiation and the possible risks associated with the image. This understanding, combined with discernment of the exceeding benefits that x rays can offer them, individuals can be in a well-informed position to evaluate the ratio between the health risks and the benefits of the test, enabling them to participate in a shared decision making with their physicians, and make evidence-based decisions in regard to their personal health. (Lumbreras et al.) With this in mind, ensuring that patients are well informed about X-rays prior to the tests themselves could result in enhancing the execution of patient treatment and diagnosis accuracy. This is a result of fewer people refusing medical imaging on the basis of misinformation, paired with a reduction of unnecessary X-ray tests given to those who are not in the need of medical imaging, despite perhaps claiming otherwise. According to Dr Maria del Rosario Perez, a scientist with the World Health Organization's Department of Public Health, "if patients are not properly informed about the risks and benefits of an imaging procedure, they may make choices that are more harmful rather than beneficial to their health" (World Health Organization). To a great degree, a well-informed patient is beneficial to not only the patient themselves but equally to medical health care providers.

To dive a little deeper into the misinformation or lack of information the many have in regard to X-rays, there are several common themes that people should have a factual understanding on prior to medical imaging tests. First of all, a study of 164 participants in Vermont concluded that "only eight percent of respondents from the general public expressed having confidence in their knowledge of ionizing radiation, indicating a great need for additional public education" (Evans et al. 2). That being the case, a great deal of the general public could be making health decisions concerning medical imaging based on factors other than factual knowledge, whether it be emotion or perception based. What's more, according to research, many individuals were unable to identify the differences in radiation dose or potential risk severity between CT scans, X-rays or MRIs. (Kumar and Irving). Overall, it is necessary for patients to be well-informed about the imaging tests they are receiving as well as the associated risks, so that individuals can include factual evidence in their health care decisions.

In the context of the general public's perception of X-ray tests, a wide scope of differing interpretations and opinions is often seen, which can also potentially have an impact on patient care. Many of the public perceptions of X-rays pertain to the associated risks. This wide scope of perceptions ranges from underestimation to overestimation to anywhere in between when it comes down to the perceived risks in association with the test. According to the Journal of Clinical Urology, within a survey of one hundred patients undergoing a variety of radiological investigations, "24% of participants perceived X-rays to have no risk" (Krewski et al. 636). On the other end of the spectrum, there are many patients refusing doctors' requests for medical imaging tests in fear of radiation and developing cancer (Oakley and Harrison), which could potentially lead to a misdiagnosis, causing complications in their treatment. With this in mind, people are clearly relying on other considerations than factual evidence to make decisions towards medical imaging, and their willingness to participate in such tests. When faced with or hearing about a medical decision, the emotions that arise or lack thereof can often impact how a situation is perceived. To give an example, "if one is faced with anxiety, pain, discomfort or other intense emotions while being faced with a medical decision such as an x ray test, these pressing emotions will often be used as information in the decision process, as well as for information processing and judgement" (Dauer et al. 757). That being said, whatever knowledge the patient had, whether factual or not, becomes at risk of being altered by how they are perceiving and reacting to various situations.

Although the general knowledge concerning medical X-rays is influenced by many factors, the public perception of these tests is impressionable in a similar fashion. In relation to the perceived risks, the journal of Human and Ecological Risk Assessment notes that public perceptions can be influenced by an array of different factors, such as media coverage, familiarity with the procedure, the level of comprehension concerning the associated risks as well as the benefits, the level of control that the patient has, as well as the severity that the risks pertain (Krewski et al. 636). That being said, the perceptions that individuals form in regard to medical X-rays can potentially derive from many different sources, or a mixture of several. For example, media coverage on X-rays and other medical imaging tests will often "exacerbate the public's concerns about health risks" (Hendee 1114), rather than offer education to the general public. One is more likely to come across news stories of X-rays going wrong, or media coverage about the adverse effects that have produced in response to an X-ray test as opposed to the simple routine procedure. Beyond that, people's perceptions are often influenced by those around them, in particular those they care about. This issue goes to say that an individual's perception of X-rays could be susceptible to being altered if someone they value has a contradicting opinion or experience with the test. As a result of how impressionable the public's perception of medical x rays is, many of these conceptions differ or contradict from current scientific findings, and could potentially affect their entire treatment plan.

That being said, the manner in which the general public perceives a certain medical imaging test such as X-rays is noteworthy, and a positive perception is important for the patient as well as the medical professional. While the knowledge and awareness of the general public on the subject of medical imaging, in particular, the dose and risk of radiation are important, the perceptions that patients hold, have an equal or greater significance (Dauer et al. 757). This is because "medical decision making is influenced by cognitive and affective responses" (Dauer et al. 757). Having knowledge on a certain procedure is of great significance, but how a person perceives the test will most likely determine their overall stance. An individual's affect "influences virtually every aspect of human functioning" (Dauer et al. 757). To elaborate, how they perceive not only the medical imaging itself, but also the interactions with their doctor, and the emotions that arise in response, could potentially impair the capacity of objective decision making, resulting in a risk of impacting their treatment plan. With this in mind, how a patient perceives an X-ray, and its associated risks could determine their willingness to receive one altogether. When the general public has a positive perception of X-ray imaging, overall treatment and diagnostic outcomes will improve, as well as patient satisfaction.

Taking into account that the knowledge and perception on X-rays vastly differs between medical professionals and the general public, one might be left wondering how to bridge this gap. While it is clear that there is a significant need for better patient education by imaging providers and medical professionals, how they decide to go about patient education is fundamental to the reinforcement of public awareness and a more positive perception of x ray tests. According to research, there are several ways in which medical professionals can communicate with patients in regard to medical imaging tests and their respective benefits and risks (Dauer, et al. 757), that can be highly effective. First of all, the journal mentions that language that doctors use and the presentation of the medical imaging test should be simplified, with a goal to convey a clear and easily comprehensible message. Numbers and visuals should be supplemented alongside the communication with the patient, to add a visual aid and to ensure comprehension. In addition, dialogue with the patient, as well as addressing any concerns or questions is crucial to developing and maintaining patient satisfaction. Lastly, patient understanding should be evaluated or observed in some way prior to the imaging test. This can be done in many ways, for example observing the patient's body language and feedback, to ensure they understand the procedure and so that they feel valued in the process of their treatment. (Dauer, et al. 757) All things considered, "good communication, care for the patient as an individual, and emotional support contribute to a positive patient experience" (Bolderston 357) and can optimize the outcome of the treatment.

In summary, the general public's knowledge and perspectives towards x-ray tests is all over the place. For the most part, patients seem to lack the necessary information needed to enable them to make objective medical decisions, such as radiation dosage and potential health risks. Additionally, people perceive the risks of x-ray tests anywhere from harmless to lethal. Overall health care professionals need to make sure that they are supporting the patient to make sure that they understand the medical imaging test and are able to weigh out the risks and benefits. Increasing patient knowledge and perception will enhance the accuracy of patient care and increase patient willingness to participate in x-rays.

CHAPTER 10

Future in improving speed, safety, and quality

Viveka Pimenta

The Evolution of CT

Computed tomography has evolved to its ubiquitous role in diagnostic imaging due to the developments made over the last few decades, helical scanning and multi-detector row CT being two of the most important. These innovations expedited the improvement of imaging speed, low-contrast detectability, and spatial resolution of 3-dimensional objects — in fact, speed has increased by over nine orders of magnitude since the 1970s. To visualize this a bit better, that means that the number of pixels generated from raw data points measured each second has risen from 10 pixels per second to 1 000 000 000 pixels per second in the last forty years, and continues to improve each year (Pelc). It is because of these innovations that computed tomography has emerged as such a widely-used diagnostic tool in medicine today, and looking at the patterns of past progression can help us predict where the development is heading next. Current and future advances in CT are driven by the need to improve the image quality and speed, reduce radiation dose, and search for ways to implement it more efficiently in clinical settings (Pelc).

Improvements in CT Scanning Speed

Imaging speed has increased by two methods: 1) reducing the time it takes to obtain data from any one of the parallel axial slices that make up the three-dimensional image, and 2) increasing how many slices are imaged at any given time via multi-detector row technology. Immediately after the inception of CT, the minimum time for a scan was sharply reduced by increasing the gantry rotation speed, and slow but steady reductions have continued since 1980 (Pelc). One attempt to increase CT speed with a short scan-time was the electron-beam CT, designed specifically for rapid cardiac imaging. However, it used a stationary detector ring, and without mechanical rotation, it was inefficient and quickly fell out of favour amongst physicians (Booji et al.).

The more commonly used dual-source scanners operate by using two X-ray sources which work concurrently with two detectors on the gantry. This halves the necessary minimum rotation so that required images can be obtained with a minimum scan time that is two times faster for each gantry rotation speed (Pelc).

Future advances in increasing CT scan speed cannot be achieved by using more than two sources, because of hardware limitations — the sizes of the detectors cannot be further reduced to fit multiple sources on the gantry without sacrificing the integrity of the scanner (Pelc). The obvious next question is then: are we able to increase the gantry's speed of rotation any further? During rotation, the centripetal force exerted on the X-ray tube and other structures attached to the rotating frame acts as a technical limitation. Developments in the 1990s allowed the gantry structures to sustain g-forces of up to forty times the earth's gravitational pull, allowing for increased acceleration and decreased rotation time. This feat of engineering continues to increase the tolerance to g-forces, and the shortest rotation time of 0.25 seconds is expected to reduce to less than 0.2 seconds in the next decade (Pelc).

These advancements have been driven by the need for clear imaging of the heart at any point in its cardiac cycle without multiple rounds of CT scanning, which exposes the patients to higher doses of radiation. By reducing imaging time, the blur resulting from the heart's motion is also reduced. Scan times of under a second allow any phase of the cardiac cycle to be imaged with higher temporal resolution and minimal radiation exposure. However, even with reducing scan time to 0.1 seconds, motion within the body still causes blurring, and while further reductions in imaging time could improve temporal resolution, other technological advancements may solve this issue (Pelc).

For example, the introduction of time delayed summation allows CT systems to support faster rotation speeds without sacrificing resolution of the images (Nowak et al.). The pixels shift throughout the scanning, orienting themselves to self-correct for detector motion. To make the best of this method, it has been advanced by fixing the focal spot position of the x-rays so that it further reduces blur. The systems are able to support an increase in gantry rotation without losing image quality from increasing the frame rate (Nowak et al.).

Future avenues for more efficient CT scanning include the development of algorithms that correct residual motion during the scanning window by estimating the heart's motion as part of the image reconstruction (Pelc). Developing this further will revolutionize cardiac imaging with reduced blurring in images and much more efficient, effective CT exams. It will also contribute to decreasing the risks posed by radiation. Over the next ten years, we could see the minimum rotation time of CT scanners reduced to around 0.15 seconds, and consequently, minimum imaging times could be as low as 0.040 seconds per image in dual-source CT systems and even 0.075 seconds in single-source CT (Pelc).

Improvements in CT Safety: Reducing Radiation Dose

Radiation doses have been steadily decreasing since the inception of computed tomography, but dose reduction has become all the more necessitated by the ever-increasing number of CT scans performed worldwide (Booji et al). Computed tomography contributes a majority of the total population's radiation dose from medical imaging, so dose reduction is a vital focus during the development of improved technologies (Palmer).

Photon counting detector technology is a promising advancement, as its purpose is to maximize efficiency of CT via high spatial resolution, energy discrimination, and primarily by economizing radiation dose, with a reduction of 80-percent so far. The goal is to reduce CT doses below 1 millisievert (Palmer). Current doses of radiation from CT can be up to 10 mSv (Center for Devices and Radiological Health).

Filters are being developed to eliminate softer energy radiation that emits from the X-rays by changing the shape of the beam so that radiation is targeted only towards the specific anatomical regions being clinically examined (Palmer). This too will limit patients' radiation dosage and maximize efficiency.

In a CT scan of the heart, the clinical implications of this development are that breast and lung tissue -- which are adjacent to the areas of clinical interest and also extremely sensitive to radiation -- will no longer be needlessly subjected to the same levels of radiation as the tissue being examined (Palmer).

Increasing specialization of CT scanners will ultimately reduce patients' exposure to radiation and, consequently, increase access to diagnostic services for high-risk populations that would most benefit from early screenings for disease.

Recent developments in specialized CT include a novel technique called cycloidal computed technology. This method not only rotates the x-rays around the patient, but also scans forwards and backwards for more volumetric coverage. Thanks to the use of beamlets, in which slitted filters break up a single X-ray beam into tiny beamlets, this new method also reduces the patient's exposure to radiation while producing a more precise image (Hagen et al.).

Optimizing the use of CT so that the patient is not exposed to too much radiation is of the utmost importance, and can also be achieved by optimizing the X-ray beam collimation and controlling the flow of X-ray energy on the subject. For example, in helical scanners, the edges of the subject cannot be reconstructed using data because they are nearly out of the system's angular range of illumination. So while radiation is being administered to all these regions, no data can be retrieved (Pelc).

Recent improvements to collimators eliminate all imaging at these extreme regions, improving radiation dose for the patients. It is important that the flow of energy from the X-rays, or illuminated flux, can be controlled. The number of photons detected in each voxel for a given view can vary between views, and controlling this variance in flux is essential to optimize efficiency of the reconstruction (Pelc). In turn, optimizing the system also improves dose regulation.

Methods of controlling this flux include modulating the X-ray tube current (measured in milliamperes or mA) by using bowtie filters to control the view angle and slice location. This creates an opportunity to specify the intensity of the X-ray beams and dispense lower levels of radiation (Pelc). The bow-tie filter method is already being improved upon with future avenues working towards increased control of X-ray beams. These advances include inverse geometry CT, which creates the bowtie virtually, and dynamic attenuators which can fine-tune the illumination pattern, radiation dose, and other parameters to the patient's specific needs (Pelc). This particular method doubles the dose efficiency, displaying an increased need for personalized medicine to be prioritized.

Another priority in the journey to reduce radiation doses is image reconstruction. It has already been advanced from the previous filtered back-projection method to the more accurate and efficient method of iterative reconstruction (Pelc). The FBP method works well with perfect raw data lacking noise, which is not always clinically practical. Its inefficiency with imperfect raw data can be overcome using iterative reconstruction, a model-based algorithm which uses statistics to reduce electronic noise and increase contrast in the reconstructed imagery (Pelc). The development of post-processing deep-learning reconstruction software to reduce image noise can also be used to maximize dose efficiency, as any noise created during scanning would not have to be corrected immediately during the examination (Steuwe et al.)

These technological improvements should be supplemented with evidence-based action from radiologists to maximize dose efficiency, namely: lowering kilovoltage, monitoring standard dose protocols for inefficiencies, comparing common dosage levels between facilities in a region to narrow the range of acceptable values, and customizing radiation dose for each clinical case (Palmer).

Improvements in CT Safety: Reducing Radiation Dose

In addition to improvements in temporal resolution and dose reduction, the spatial resolution of CT scanners has been improving and shows potential for improving further. This is achieved by advancing the detector technology. Reducing the aperture of the detectors improves the spatial resolution of the CT scanner, and from 1975 to 2015, the detector aperture has been reduced from 1.3 mm2 to just under 0.4 mm2. This reduction can be attributed to diminishing the thickness of the minimum slice CT can take, by reducing the axial or slice direction of the detector (Pelc).

While detector development seemingly skyrocketed immediately following the genesis of CT, there has been little to no development in this area since the 1980s. Scintillator photodiode detectors have been commonly in use since that time, where X-rays are absorbed in the scintillator and produce detectable light which the photodiode can convert into electrical signals. Typically these detectors are spaced 1 mm apart and their reflectors are about 0.1 mm in thickness, and the current geometric efficiency of the detectors in two dimensions is about 80% (Pelc). Detection at a higher resolution could potentially be possible with smaller scintillators if the hardware limitations in constructing the small devices could be overcome. However, there is a technical limitation; the proportions of these detectors would force the reflectors to take up more space on the detector surface and reduce geometric efficiency, making the improvement null. The dose efficiency would also be reduced with the diminished quality of the detectors. The difficulties with scintillator photodiode detectors have put a damper on the technological progression of detector aperture over the last several decades (Pelc).

If aperture could be improved, both clearer imaging and dose reduction would be obtained. The mid to high spatial frequencies of the smaller aperture could reduce the "white noise" produced by the detectors themselves, improving image quality and accuracy of the CT scanner so that small signals can be distinguished from each other even at very near proximity. Electronic noise obscures the signal to be detected and limits the measurement quality. Current CT scanners can only overcome this limitation by increasing the radiation dose to increase the signal, which is something to be avoided (Pelc).

A promising development in the technology is the direct conversion photon-counting detector, which utilizes each photon to create charge carriers that follow parallel electric field lines in the semiconductor (Pelc). The electric field lines, which are proportionate to the amount of charge being carried, never intersect, and this eliminates the need for reflectors, which typically minimize unfavourable electronic interactions between circuits. Removing reflectors removes all the geometric inefficiency of the scintillator photodiode detectors, and thus direct conversion photon-counting detectors have a significantly higher quality of spatial resolution. The direct conversion photon-counting detectors also detect and count X-ray photons to eliminate the issue of electronic noise. All it requires is setting a threshold in a certain energy range to limit noise signals produced by low-energy photons and only process the photons above that threshold (Pelc). Direct conversion photon-counting detectors not only have 100% geometric efficiency; they also avoid the issues of electronic noise altogether and produce images with much higher spatial resolution (Pelc).

However, these direct conversion photon-counting detectors require further research and development to improve beyond their technical limitations before becoming mainstream. These limitations include the count rate of the current systems. The current capability of the photon counters is insufficient for sustaining the magnitude of energy from X-rays on the detector over prolonged use, and this slows down the imaging speed to compensate. Consistently pushing the detectors to their photon-counting limits may also cause a "pulse pile-up" in which the information becomes distorted (Pelc).

It is expected to take a few years before they become readily available. In addition, due to the high cost of the detectors, they cannot be marketed as general diagnostic imaging tools for speedy, large surface area detection. They are designed for systems that prioritize image clarity and dose efficiency, and will thus be rolled out for specialized CT scanning (Pelc).

Conclusion: Future Direction of CT Innovation in Speed, Safety, and Quality

The journey to develop computed tomography technology that utilizes low doses of radiation to deliver speedy scans with highly accurate, detailed images will continue for as long as technology continues to advance.

Temporal resolution continues to evolve by reducing scan times and increasing gantry rotation speeds. These benefits are amplified with the use of dual-source scanners and advanced reconstruction algorithms which account for the blur attributed to motion (Pelc).

The future of computed tomography includes CT systems which can operate more efficiently on reduced dosage, detecting smaller abnormalities earlier in the disease progression. It includes scanners that are faster, fully automated, and intuitive to use with set parameters for each type of CT scan and alarms that alert physicians to radiation dosage levels crossing a certain threshold (Loria). Methods that improve image quality for CT also contribute heavily to dose reduction. Highly efficient photon-counting detectors with decreased apertures and advanced iterative reconstruction methods play an important role in dose reduction as well (Pelc). With the increasing popularity of photon-counting detectors and dual source CT, future avenues for advancement could lie within developing a hybrid of the two to maximize system efficiency (Sawall et al.).

The development of dose-efficient CT systems in the future could involve removing image noise with deep-learning based reconstruction software, which improves further upon iterative reconstruction (Steuwe et al.). The quality of computed tomography would also benefit from improving the interpretation of the data from a CT scan by developing a computer-based design with increased analytics for simpler diagnostics and a more efficient user interface for clinical settings (Loria).

Multiple specialized systems will be needed to implement all the improvements CT is facing in the upcoming decade (Pelc). Speed, safety, and quality of imaging are all driving the development to a more efficient and personalized CT delivery that is accessible to all. With such an incredible diversity of technological advances in diagnostic imaging, personalized patient care will be easier than ever before.

Works Cited

"About the ACR AC." American College of Radiology, www.acr.org/Clinical-Resources/ACR- Appropriateness-Criteria/About-the-ACR-A

Adams, Judith E., et al. "Radiology." Pediatric Bone, Elsevier Inc., 2012, pp. 277–307, doi:10.1016/B978-0-12-382040-2.10012-7.

"A Gentleman's Crazy Idea." History of CT (Computed Tomography), Siemens Healthineers MedMuseum, www.medmuseum.siemens-healthineers.com/en/stories-from-the-museum/history-of-ct. Accessed May 6 2021. IN TEXT: ("A Gentleman's Crazy Idea")

Allan M. Cormack – Biographical. NobelPrize.org. Nobel Media AB 2021. Accessed 3 May 2021, https://www.nobelprize.org/prizes/medicine/1979/cormack/biographical/ IN TEXT: (Allan M. Cormack – Biographical)

Bajoghli, Morteza et al. "Children, CT Scan and Radiation." International journal of preventive medicine vol. 1,4 (2010): 220-2.

Baldwin, J., and V. Grantham. "Radiation Hormesis: Historical and Current Perspectives." Journal of Nuclear Medicine Technology, vol. 43, no. 4, 2015, pp. 242–46. Crossref, doi:10.2967/jnmt.115.166074.

Baranauckas, Carla. "William H. Oldendorf, 67, Dies; Developed X-ray Imaging Device." The New York Times, 1 Jan. 1993, p. 20, www.nytimes.com/1993/01/01/obituaries/william-h-oldendorf-67-dies-developed-X-ray-imaging-device.html. IN TEXT: (Baranauckas, 20)

Beatty, Jean. "The Radon Transform and the Mathematics of Medical Imaging." The Radon Transform and the Mathematics of Medical Imaging - Honors Thesis Paper 646, Colby College, Digital Commons @ Colby, 2012, digitalcommons.colby.edu/cgi/viewcontent.cgi?article=1649&context=honorstheses.   IN TEXT: (Beatty 10)

Bell, Daniel J. "X-ray Tube: Radiology Reference Article." Radiopaedia, Jan. 2021, radiopaedia.org/articles/X-ray-tube-1.

Berdahl, Carl T., et al. "Emergency Department Computed Tomography Utilization in the United States and Canada." Annals of Emergency Medicine, vol. 62, no. 5, 2013, pp. 496–494.e3., doi:10.1016/j.annemergmed.2013.02.018.

Bhattacharyya, Kalyan. "Godfrey Newbold Hounsfield (1919-2004): The Man Who Revolutionized Neuroimaging." Annals of Indian Academy of Neurology, vol. 19, no. 4, Medknow Publications, 1 Oct. 2016, pp. 448–50, doi:10.4103/0972-2327.194414.

Bolderston, Amanda. "Patient Experience in Medical Imaging and Radiation Therapy." Journal of Medical Imaging and Radiation Sciences, vol. 47, no. 4, 2016, pp. 356–61. Crossref, doi:10.1016/j.jmir.2016.09.002.

Booji, Ronald, et al. "Technological Developments of X-Ray Computed Tomography over Half a Century: User's Influence on Protocol Optimization." European Journal of Radiology, vol. 131, 1 Oct. 2020, p. 109261, https://www.ejradiology.com/article/S0720-048X(20)30450-2/fulltext, 10.1016/j.ejrad.2020.109261. Accessed 10 Dec. 2020.

Bosch de Basea, Magda, et al. "Trends and Patterns in the Use of Computed Tomography in Children and Young Adults in Catalonia — Results from the EPI-CT Study." Pediatric Radiology, vol. 46, no. 1, 2015, pp. 119–129., doi:10.1007/s00247-015-3434-5.

Boston Children's Hospital. "CT Scan." Boston Children's Hospital, 2021, www.childrenshospital.org/conditions-and-treatments/treatments/ct-scan

Brenner, David J., and Eric J. Hall. "Cancer Risks from CT Scans: Now We Have Data, What Next?" Radiology, vol. 265, no. 2, 2012, pp. 330–331., doi:10.1148/radiol.12121248.

Brenner, David J., and Eric J. Hall. "Computed Tomography — An Increasing Source of Radiation Exposure." New England Journal of Medicine, vol. 357, no. 22, 2007, pp. 2277–2284., doi:10.1056/nejmra072149.

Britannica, The Editors of Encyclopaedia. "Allan MacLeod Cormack". Encyclopedia Britannica, 20 Jul. 1998, https://www.britannica.com/biography/Allan-MacLeod-Cormack. Accessed 4 May, 2021. IN TEXT: (Britannica, 1998)

Britannica, The Editors of Encyclopaedia. "Computed tomography". Encyclopedia Britannica, 26 Jan. 2012, https://www.britannica.com/topic/computed-tomography. Accessed 2 May 2021.   IN TEXT: (Britannica, 2012)

Bulas, Dorothy I., et al. "Image Gently: Why We Should Talk to Parents About CT in Children." American Journal of Roentgenology, vol. 192, no. 5, 2009, pp. 1176–1178., doi:10.2214/ajr.08.2218.

Burgio, Ernesto et al. "Ionizing Radiation and Human Health: Reviewing Models of Exposure and Mechanisms of Cellular Damage. An Epigenetic Perspective." International journal of environmental research and public health vol. 15,9 1971. 10 Sep. 2018, doi:10.3390/ijerph15091971"Computed Tomography (Ct) Scans and Cancer Fact Sheet." National Cancer Institute, 14 Aug. 2019, www.cancer.gov/about-cancer/diagnosis-staging/ct-scans-factsheet.

Cassoobhoy, Arefa. "CT Scan (CAT Scan): Purpose, Procedure, Risks, Side-Effects, Results." WebMD, WebMD LLC, 13 Dec. 2020, www.webmd.com/cancer/what-is-a-ct-scan#:~:text=CT%20scans%20can%20detect%20bone,caused%20by%20a%20car%20accident.

Center for Devices and Radiological Health. "What Are the Radiation Risks from CT?" U.S. Food and Drug Administration, FDA, www.fda.gov/radiation-emitting-products/medical-X-ray-imaging/what-are-radiation-risks-ct.

Center for Devices and Radiological Health. What Is Computed Tomography?: Fda. www.fda.gov/radiation-emitting-products/medical-X-ray-imaging/what-computed-tomography#xray.

"Computed Tomography (CT)." National Institute of Biomedical Imaging and Bioengineering (NIBIB), www.nibib.nih.gov/science-education/science-topics/computed-tomography-ct.

"Computed Tomography (CT or CAT) Scan of the Bones." Johns Hopkins Medicine, The Johns Hopkins University, The Johns Hopkins Hospital, and Johns Hopkins Health System., www.hopkinsmedicine.org/health/treatment-tests-and-therapies/computed-tomography-ct-or-cat-scan-of-the-bones.

Cook Children's. "Computed Tomography (CT): Radiology." Cook Children's Health Care System, 2021, cookchildrens.org/radiology/specialty-programs/Pages/computed-tomography.aspx.

Crownover, Brian K, and Jennifer L Bepko. "Appropriate and safe use of diagnostic imaging." American family physician vol. 87,7 (2013): 494-501

CT Scan Versus MRI Versud X-RAY: What Type of Imaging Do I Need? www.hopkinsmedicine.org/health/treatment-tests-and-therapies/ct-vs-mri-vs-xray.

Dauer, Lawrence T., et al. "Fears, Feelings, and Facts: Interactively Communicating Benefits and Risks of Medical Radiation With Patients." American Journal of Roentgenology, vol. 196, no. 4, 2011, pp. 756–61. Crossref, doi:10.2214/ajr.10.5956.

Davis, Lawrence M. "CT Scan (CAT Scan) Procedure Side Effects, Purpose, CT vs. MRI." Edited by William C. Shiel, EMedicineHealth, WebMD, Inc., 9 Oct. 2019, www.emedicinehealth.com/ct_scan/article_em.htm.

DenOtter, Tami D., and Johanna Schubert. "Hounsfield Unit." Definitions, Qeios, 2020, doi:10.32388/aavabi.

"Diagnosing Muscle and Bone Disorders With CT Scans." Envision Radiology, 18 Jan. 2021, www.envrad.com/diagnosing-muscle-and-bone-disorders-with-ct-scans/.

"Differences Between X-rays, CT Scans & MRI's." Envision Radiology, 30 Mar. 2021, www.envrad.com/difference-between-X-ray-ct-scan-and-mri/#:~:text=Doctors%20 use%20x%2Drays%20to,the%20structure%20and%20a%20computer.&text=x-%2Dray%20images%20are%20in,CT%20scan%20images%20are%203D. Accessed 7 May, 2021. IN TEXT: ("Differences Between X-rays, CT Scans, & MRI's")

Evans, Katherine M., et al. "An Exploratory Analysis of Public Awareness and Perception of Ionizing Radiation and Guide to Public Health Practice in Vermont." Journal of Environmental and Public Health, vol. 2015, 2015, pp. 1–6. Crossref, doi:10.1155/2015/476495.

Fayad, Laura Marie. CT Scan Versus MRI Versus X-ray: What Type of Imaging Do I Need? https://www.hopkinsmedicine.org/health/treatment-tests-and-therapies/ct-vs-mri-vs-X-ray. Accessed 7 May 2021.

Freudenberg, L. S., and T. Beyer. "Subjective Perception of Radiation Risk." Journal of Nuclear Medicine, vol. 52, no. Supplement_2, 2011, pp. 29S-35S. Crossref, doi:10.2967/jnumed.110.085720.

Frush, Karen. "Image gently: is overuse of CT scans in the ED harming our children?" Contemporary Pediatrics, vol. 28, no. 11, 2011, p. 24-32. Gale Academic OneFile, link.gale.com/apps/doc/A456582288/AONE?u=uniwater&sid=AONE&xid=04155c20. Accessed 7 May 2021.

Goldman, L. W. "Principles of CT and CT Technology." Journal of Nuclear Medicine Technology, vol. 35, no. 3, Sept. 2007, pp. 115–128., doi:10.2967/jnmt.107.042978.

Goldman, L. W. "Principles of CT: Radiation Dose and Image Quality." Journal of Nuclear Medicine Technology, vol. 35, no. 4, Dec. 2007, pp. 213–225., doi:10.2967/jnmt.106.037846.

Goske, M J. "Doctor, Is a CT Scan Safe for My Child?" The British Journal of Radiology, vol. 87, no. 1034, 2014, p. 20130517., doi:10.1259/bjr.20130517.

Goske, Marilyn J., et al. "The Image Gently Campaign: Working Together to Change Practice." American Journal of Roentgenology, vol. 190, no. 2, 2008, pp. 273–274., doi:10.2214/ajr.07.3526.

Greenburg, Jack O. "William Henry Oldendorf - A Tribute ." Journal of Neuroimaging, 1993, pp. 148–149., www.asnweb.org/i4a/pages/index.cfm?pageID=3329. IN TEXT: (Greenburg 148-149)

Hacking, Craig, and Behrang Amini. "Hodgkin Lymphoma: Radiology Reference Article." Radiopaedia Blog RSS, Radiopaedia.org, radiopaedia.org/articles/hodgkin-lymphoma.

Hagen, Charlotte K., et al. "Cycloidal Computed Tomography." Physical Review Applied, vol. 14, no. 1, 23 July 2020, 10.1103/physrevapplied.14.014069. Accessed 22 Sept. 2020.

Harmonay, Vikki. "It's All About CT Detectors." Atlantis Worldwide, 2 Dec. 2020, info.atlantisworldwide.com/blog/its-all-about-ct-detectors.

Hendee, W. R. "Personal and Public Perceptions of Radiation Risks." RadioGraphics, vol. 11, no. 6, 1991, pp. 1109–19. Crossref, doi:10.1148/radiographics.11.6.1749852.

Hendee, William R., et al. "Addressing Overutilization in Medical Imaging." Radiology, vol. 257, no. 1, 1 Oct. 2010, pp. 240–245., doi:10.1148/radiol.10100063.

"History of Medicine: Dr. Roentgen's Accidental X-rays." Columbia University Department of Surgery, columbiasurgery.org/news/2015/09/17/history-medicine-dr-roentgen-s-accidental-X-rays#:~:text=Wilhelm%20Roentgen%2C%20Professor%20of%20Physics,rays%20could%20pass%20through%20glass.&text=Because%20he%20

did%20not%20know,meaning%20'unknown%2C'%20rays. Accessed 7 May, 2021. IN TEXT: ("History of Medicine: Dr Roentgen's Accidental X-rays")

History of the CT Scan | Catalina Imaging. https://catalinaimaging.com/history-ct-scan/. Accessed 8 May 2021.

Hounsfield Unit | Radiology Reference Article | Radiopaedia.Org. https://radiopaedia. org/articles/hounsfield-unit. Accessed 8 May 2021.

Hounsfield, Godfrey N. "Computed Medical Imaging." Medical Physics, vol. 7, no. 4, 1980, pp. 283–90, doi:10.1118/1.594709.

"Johann Radon Formulates the Basis for Computed Tomography." Johann Radon Formulates the Basis for Computed Tomography : History of Information, www.historyofinformation.com/detail.php?id=579. IN TEXT: ("Johann Radon Formulates the Basis for Computed Tomography")

Kak, A. C., and Malcolm Slaney. Principles of Computerized Tomographic Imaging. IEEE Press, 1988, https://www.slaney.org/pct/pct-toc.html.

Khurshid, S. J., and A. M. Hussain. "Nuclear Magnetic Resonance Imaging (MRI)." JPMA. The Journal of the Pakistan Medical Association, vol. 41, no. 10, J Pak Med Assoc, 1991, pp. 259–64, doi:10.1007/978-0-387-79061-9_5338.

Klopfenstein, Bethany J., et al. "Comparison of 3 T MRI and CT for the Measurement of Visceral and Subcutaneous Adipose Tissue in Humans." British Journal of Radiology, vol. 85, no. 1018, British Institute of Radiology, Oct. 2012, p. e826, doi:10.1259/bjr/57987644.

Knott, Laurence. "CT Scan." Edited by Helen Huins, Patient.info, Patient Platform Limited., 18 July 2018, patient.info/treatment-medication/ct-scan.

Krewski, Daniel, et al. "Public Perception of Population Health Risks in Canada: Health Hazards and Sources of Information." Human and Ecological Risk Assessment: An International Journal, vol. 12, no. 4, 2006, pp. 626–44. Crossref, doi:10.1080/10807030600561832.

Kumar, Prakrit R., and Stuart Irving. "Patients' Perception of Radiation Safety of Radiological Investigations in Urology." Journal of Clinical Urology, 2020. Crossref, doi:10.1177/2051415820964979.

Kutanzi, Kristy R et al. "Pediatric Exposures to Ionizing Radiation: Carcinogenic Considerations." International journal of environmental research and public health vol. 13,11 1057. 28 Oct. 2016, doi:10.3390/ijerph13111057

Lell, Michael, M., et al. "Evolution in Computed Tomography". Investigative Radiology, vol. 50, no. 9, September 2015, pp. 629–644. doi: 10.1097/RLI.0000000000000172. IN TEXT: (Lell et al. 629-644)

Lin, Eugene, and Adam Alessio. "What Are the Basic Concepts of Temporal, Contrast, and Spatial Resolution in Cardiac CT?" Journal of Cardiovascular Computed Tomography, vol. 3, no. 6, 30 July 2009, pp. 403–408., doi:10.1016/j.jcct.2009.07.003.

Loria, Kieth. "What's next in CT Technology." Radiology Today Magazine, Great Valley Publishing, Apr. 2016, What's Next in CT Technology. Accessed 7 May 2021.

Lumbreras, Blanca, et al. "Avoiding Fears and Promoting Shared Decision-Making: How Should Physicians Inform Patients about Radiation Exposure from Imaging Tests?" PLOS ONE, edited by Eugenio Paci, vol. 12, no. 7, 2017, p. e0180592. Crossref, doi:10.1371/journal.pone.0180592.

Mathews, John D, et al. "Cancer Risk in 680 000 People Exposed to Computed Tomography Scans in Childhood or Adolescence: Data Linkage Study of 11 Million Australians." The BMJ, British Medical Journal Publishing Group, 21 May 2013, www.bmj.com/content/346/bmj.f2360.

Mayo Clinic. CT Scan. https://www.mayoclinic.org/tests-procedures/ct-scan/about/pac-20393675. Accessed 4 May 2021.

Mazziotta, John, C., and Robert C. Collins. "William H. Oldendorf, M.D. (1925–1992)". Journal of Computer Assisted Tomography, vol. 17, no. 2, March-April 1993, pp. 169–170.   IN TEXT: (Mazziotta et al. 169-170)

McCollough, Cynthia H., et al. "Answers to Common Questions About the Use and Safety of CT Scans." Mayo Clinic, www.mayoclinicproceedings.org/article/S0025-6196(15)00591-1/pdf.

National Research Council. "Health Risks from Exposure to Low Levels of Ionizing Radiation." 2006, doi:10.17226/9526.

New York State Department of Health. "What Parents Should Know About CT Scans for Children. Medical Radiation Safety, 2021, https://www.health.ny.gov/environmental/radiological/radiation_safety_guides/docs/ct_scans_children.pdf

"Nonspecific Interstitial Pneumonia (NSIP): What Is It, Causes and Treatment." Cleveland Clinic, Cleveland Clinic, 10 Nov. 2020, my.clevelandclinic.org/health/diseases/14804-nonspecific-interstitial-pneumonia-nsip#:~:text=Nonspecific%20interstitial%20pneumonia%20(NSIP)%20is%20a%20rare%20disorder%20that%20affects,the%20lungs%20and%20the%20bloodstream.

Nowak, Tristan, et al. "Time-Delayed Summation as a Means of Improving Resolution on Fast Rotating Computed Tomography Systems." Medical Physics, vol. 39, no. 4, 3 Apr. 2012, pp. 2249–2260, 10.1118/1.3697533. Accessed 9 May 2021.

Oakley, Paul A., and Deed E. Harrison. "X-ray Hesitancy: Patients' Radiophobic Concerns Over Medical X-rays." Dose-Response, vol. 18, no. 3, 2020. Crossref, doi:10.1177/1559325820959542.

Old, Jerry L., et al. "Imaging for Suspected Appendicitis." American Family Physician, vol. 71, no. 1, 1 Jan. 2005, pp. 71–78.

Oren, Ohad, et al. "Curbing Unnecessary and Wasted Diagnostic Imaging." JAMA - Journal of the American Medical Association, vol. 321, no. 3, American Medical Association, 22 Jan. 2019, pp. 245–46, doi:10.1001/jama.2018.20295.

Orrison Jr, William W, and John A Sanders. "Backprojection." Backprojection - an Overview I ScienceDirect Topics, 1995, www.sciencedirect.com/topics/engineering/backprojection. IN TEXT: (Orrison Jr and Sanders)

Palmer, Whitney J. "CT's Future: What's New in Dose Reduction." Diagnostic Imaging, MJH Life Sciences, 28 Jan. 2020, www.diagnosticimaging.com/view/cts-future-whats-new-dose-reduction.

"Patients' Perception of Radiation Safety of Radiological Investigations in Urology." Journal of Clinical Urology, 2020. Crossref, doi:10.1177/2051415820964979.

Pearce, Mark S, et al. "CT Scans in Childhood and Risk of Leukaemia and Brain Tumours – Authors' Reply." The Lancet, vol. 380, no. 9855, 2012, pp. 1736–1737., doi:10.1016/s0140-6736(12)61984-9.

Pearce, Mark S, et al. "Radiation Exposure from CT Scans in Childhood and Subsequent Risk of Leukaemia and Brain Tumours: a Retrospective Cohort Study." The Lancet, vol. 380, no. 9840, 2012, pp. 499–505., doi:10.1016/s0140-6736(12)60815-0.

Pelc, Norbert J. "Recent and Future Directions in CT Imaging." Annals of Biomedical Engineering, vol. 42, no. 2, 17 Jan. 2014, pp. 260–268, 10.1007/s10439-014-0974-z.

"Public Perception of Population Health Risks in Canada: Health Hazards and Sources of Information." Human and Ecological Risk Assessment: An International Journal, vol. 12, no. 4, 2006, pp. 626–44. Crossref, doi:10.1080/10807030600561832.

Puiu, Tibi. "What Exactly Is a Photon? Definition, Properties, Facts." ZME Science, 28 Jan. 2021, www.zmescience.com/science/what-is-photon-definition-04322/. IN TEXT: (Puiu)

"Radiation Risk from Medical Imaging." Harvard Health Publishing, Harvard Medical School, Oct. 2010, www.health.harvard.edu/cancer/radiation-risk-from-medical-imaging.

Radiology Info. "Children's (Pediatric) CT (Computed Tomography)." Radiologyinfo. org, RadiologyInfo.org, 15 May 2019, www.radiologyinfo.org/en/info/pedia-ct.

Radon, Johann. Complete Dictionary of Scientific Biography. Encyclopedia.com. 16 Apr. 2021."Encyclopedia.com, Encyclopedia.com, Accessed 6 May 2021, www.encyclopedia.com/science/dictionaries-thesauruses-pictures-and-press-releases/radon-johann. IN TEXT: ("Radon, Johann, Complete Dictionary")

Redberg, Rita F., and Rebecca Smith-bindman. "We Are Giving Ourselves Cancer." The New York Times, 31 Jan. 2014, www.nytimes.com/2014/01/31/opinion/we-are-giving- ourselves-cancer.html.

Ribeiro, Ana S. F., et al. "Radiation Exposure Awareness from Patients Undergoing Nuclear Medicine Diagnostic 99mTc-MDP Bone Scans and 2-Deoxy-2-(18F) Fluoro-D-Glucose PET/Computed Tomography Scans." Nuclear Medicine Communications, vol. 41, no. 6, 2020, pp. 582–88. Crossref, doi:10.1097/mnm.0000000000001177.

Richmond, Caroline. "Sir Godfrey Hounsfield." BMJ : British Medical Journal, vol. 329, no. 7467, BMJ Publishing Group, 2004, p. 687, /pmc/articles/PMC517662/.

Robbins, Elizabeth. "Radiation Risks from Imaging Studies in Children with Cancer." Pediatric Blood & Cancer, vol. 51, no. 4, 2008, pp. 453–457., doi:10.1002/pbc.21599.

Rubin, Geoffrey D. "Computed Tomography: Revolutionizing the Practice of Medicine for 40 Years." Radiology, vol. 273, no. 2, Radiological Society of North America Inc., 1 Nov. 2014, pp. S45–74, doi:10.1148/radiol.14141356.

Safety Commission, Canadian Nuclear. "Radiation Doses." Canadian Nuclear Safety Commission, 22 Dec. 2020, nuclearsafety.gc.ca/eng/resources/radiation/introduction-to-radiation/radiation-doses.cfm.

Sawall, S., et al. "Threshold-Dependent Iodine Imaging and Spectral Separation in a Whole-Body Photon-Counting CT System." European Radiology, 13 Mar. 2021, 10.1007/s00330-021-07786-0. Accessed 9 May 2021.

Schwartz, David T. "Counter-Point: are we really ordering too many CT scans?." The western journal of emergency medicine vol. 9,2 (2008): 120-2.

"Scientist Discovers X-rays." History.com, A&E Television Networks, 24 Nov. 2009, www.history.com/this-day-in-history/german-scientist-discovers-X-rays. Accessed 6 May 2021. IN TEXT: ("Scientist Discovers X-rays")

SickKids Staff. "CT Scan." SickKids AboutKidsHealth, 2015, www.aboutkidshealth.ca/Article?contentid=1272&language=English.

Steuwe, Andrea, et al. "Influence of a Novel Deep-Learning Based Reconstruction Software on the Objective and Subjective Image Quality in Low-Dose Abdominal Computed Tomography." The British Journal of Radiology, vol. 94, no. 1117, 1 Jan. 2021, p. 20200677, 10.1259/bjr.20200677. Accessed 9 May 2021.

Tagell, Laura, et al. "Thigh Burn – A Magnetic Resonance Imaging (MRI) Related Adverse Event." Radiology Case Reports, vol. 15, no. 12, Elsevier Inc., Dec. 2020, pp. 2569–71, doi:10.1016/j.radcr.2020.09.046.

Tan, SY, and PS Poole. "Allan MacLeod Cormack (1924–1998): Discoverer of Computerised Axial Tomography." Singapore Medical Journal, vol. 61, no. 1, 2020, pp. 4–5., doi:10.11622/smedj.2020003. IN TEXT: (Tan and Poole, 4-5)

Technical Fundamentals of Radiology and CT, by Cervantes Avendaño Guillermo, IOP Publishing, 2016, pp. 21–1-21–11.

The Eclectic History of Medical Imaging | Imaging Technology News. https://www. itnonline.com/article/eclectic-history-medical-imaging. Accessed 8 May 2021.

Vaughan, C.L. "Imagining the Elephant: A Biography of Allan MacLeod Cormack." American Journal of Neuroradiology, vol. 30, no. 8, 2009, doi:10.3174/ajnr.a1668. IN TEXT: (Vaughan)

"Visualizing the Body." Science Museum, Science Museum Group Collection, 30 July 2019, www.sciencemuseum.org.uk/objects-and-stories/medicine/visualis-ing-body#body-scanning-technologies. Accessed May 6 2021. IN TEXT: ("Visualizing the Body")

Waldman, Steven D. "Computed Tomography." Pain Review, Elsevier, 2009, p. 366, doi:10.1016/B978-1-4160-5893-9.00217-3.

Wininger, Kevin L. "On the Foundations of X-ray Computed Tomography in Medicine: A Fundamental Review of the 'Radon Transform' and a Tribute to Johann Radon." Maa. org, 16 Mar. 2012, www.maa.org/sites/default/files/images/upload_library/46/HOM-SIGMAA2012/JRadonTransform_Wininger.pdf. IN TEXT: (Wininger)

Withers, Philip J., et al. "X-ray Computed Tomography." Nature Reviews Methods Primers, vol. 1, no. 1, Nature Publishing Group, Dec. 2021, p. 18, doi:10.1038/s43586-021-00015-4.

Wolpert, Samuel M. "Neuroradiology Classics." American Journal of Neuroradiology, vol. 21, no. 3, 1 Mar. 2000, pp. 605–606. IN TEXT: (Wolpert 605-606)

World Health Organization. "Communicating Radiation Risks in Pediatric Imaging". Information to support healthcare discussions about benefit and risk, 2016, https://www. who.int/ionizing_radiation/pub_meet/radiation-risks-paediatric-imaging/en/

World Health Organization. "To X-ray or Not to X-ray?" World Health Organization, 14 Apr. 2016, www.who.int/news-room/feature-stories/detail/to-X-ray-or-not-to-X-ray-.

Yu, Lifeng et al. "Radiation dose reduction in computed tomography: techniques and future perspective." Imaging in medicine vol. 1,1 (2009): 65-84. doi:10.2217/iim.09.5

Zezo. "Imaging Principles in Computed Tomography." Radiology Key, 20 Aug. 2019, radiologykey.com/imaging-principles-in-computed-tomography-2/.